S.O.S
HORMONAL
Toxics

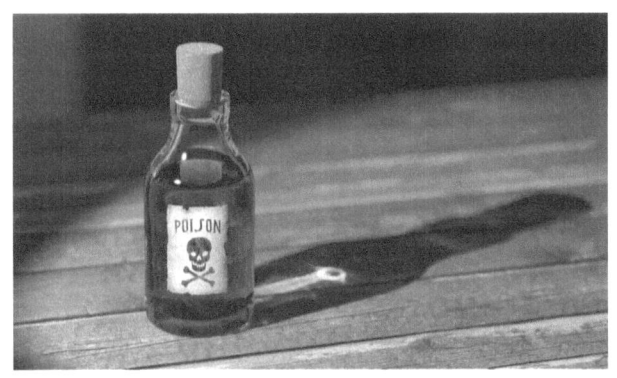

Dr. Mario Vega Carbó
Endocrinologist

First Edition, 2020

1

Table of Contents

Introduction..4

Part I. Toxic. General Aspects....................................7

Chapter 1. In the middle of a world of chemicals... 8

Part II The most common hormonal toxins...16

Chapter 2. Polychlorinated Biphenyl - PCBs 17

Chapter 3. Polychlorinated Dioxins...............................19

Chapter 4. Organochlorine pesticides 22

Chapter 5. Perfluorinated substances.............................25

Chapter 6. Phthalates 27

Chapter 7. Bisphenol-A 29

Chapter 8. Parabens 31

Chapter 9. Triclosan...33

Chapter 10. Musks 35

Chapter 11. Ultraviolet filters 37

Chapter 12. Organophosphorus pesticides.....................39

Chapter 13. Tributyltin 41

Chapter 14. Solvents and aliphenols..............................43

Chapter 15. Styrene..45

Chapter 16. Chlorinated paraffins..................................47

Chapter 17. Lead...49

Chapter 18. Cadmium 52

Chapter 19. Nickel 54

Chapter 20. Mercury 57

Chapter 21. Arsenic 59

Part III Effects on human health..................61

Chapter 22. Obesity 62

Chapter 23. Metabolic syndrome....................................66

Chapter 24. Type 1 diabetes 69

Chapter 25. Type 2 diabetes 73

Chapter 26. Hypothyroidism...76

Chapter 27. Thyroid Cancer..................................80
Chapter 28. Breast Cancer 83
Chapter 29. Polycystic ovary syndrome 86
Chapter 30. Early ovarian failure.................................89
Chapter 31. Ovarian Cancer..................................92
Chapter 32. Female infertility 95
Chapter 33. Endometriosis..................................98
Chapter 34. Uterine Fibroids 101
Chapter 35. Recurring abortions 104
Chapter 36. Intrauterine growth retardation 107
Chapter 37. Preterm Birth..................................110
Chapter 38. Low birth weight 113
Chapter 39. Early loom 116
Chapter 40. Precocious female puberty 119
Chapter 41. Small penis 123
Chapter 42. Cryptorchidism..................................126
Chapter 43. Hypospadias 129
Chapter 44. Pubertal Gynecomastia..........................132
Chapter 45. Male Infertility 135
Chapter 46. Testicular Cancer 138
Chapter 47. Prostate Cancer..................................141
Chapter 48. Autism 144
Part IV Conclusions....................................147
Chapter 49. My preventive recommendations to minimize pollution..................................148
Epilogue..15
0
Bibliographic references.........................153
About   the author...........................159
Synopsis..16
0

Introduction

We live with them daily. They are present in the air, on land, in water, in beverages, in food, in cleaning and personal hygiene items, and in thousands of other products. Worst of all is that, without our knowledge, they seriously affect our body, our health, and also that of our children.

We are talking about endocrine disruptors, a series of chemical or biological substances, usually produced by man, that alter the glands responsible for the natural secretion of hormones that regulate our body. These "imperceptible" pollutants can seriously compromise people's health and the ecological balance of the entire environment.

Endocrine disruptors can cause neurological and behavioral changes, interfere with thyroid functioning, affect reproductive health, weaken the immune system and alter sexual development, among other consequences. In addition, it can increase the risks of diabetes, obesity and certain types of cancer.

To learn more about this topic, Dr. Mario Vega Carbó, a specialist in endocrinology, presents in his first edition, SOS Hormonal Toxics, an informative resource that will educate the population on a subject as important as worrying, with which we are constantly interaction.

Divided into four sections ranging from generalities, toxic substances, health effects, and conclusions; It is a quick reading book, with clear and simple language, for the instruction of all types of audiences.

The first part of the text defines endocrine disruptors as substances capable of altering the hormonal balance and regulation of embryonic development, which can cause harmful effects on health. They can interfere, increase, block or decrease the chemical signals of hormones, sending confusing messages to the body and generating diverse consequences, such as disorders related to the reproductive health of women (breast and vagina cancer, infertility, ovarian cysts , endometriosis, spontaneous abortions, polycystic ovary syndrome, precocious puberty, among some examples), with male reproductive function (prostate and testicular cancer, decreased semen quality, infertility, cryptorchidism, congenital malformations), as well as complications metabolic that compromise the quality of life of people (metabolic syndrome, diabetes, obesity).

On the other hand, the nervous system is also one of the targets of endocrine disruptors. From neurological disorders during embryonic development to psychiatric and neurological diseases (behavioral changes, attention deficit hyperactivity disorder, reduced ability to manage stress, aggressiveness, autism, Parkinson's) have a strong environmental component influenced by these dangerous contaminants.

This book focuses on exposing the influences and alterations caused by the so-called endocrine disruptors on the glands of the body; The reader will be able to know the alterations in the thyroid function, anomalies in the reproductive tracts, sexual deviations and cardiovascular disorders, among other related health conditions, as well as the sequelae and impacts on the person and in the next generations.

This text proposes to offer the appropriate knowledge to raise awareness in relation to the serious problem that environmental toxins represent for health, as well as arouse interest in developing prevention measures at all levels of action. You are invited to take a step forward for your health and care through the reading of *"SOS. Hormonal toxins "*

Part I. Toxic. General features

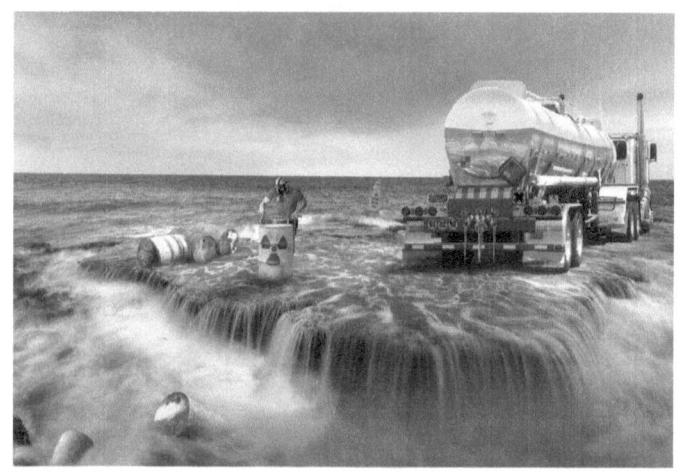

Chapter 1. In the middle of a world of chemists

If we gathered ten people of different ages and professions in the room where you are right now, each one of them could talk to you about a different issue of environmental pollution and in your sure facial expression you would see recognition.

Pollution is a subject that does not escape anyone's compression, since our pre-school stage we have heard about the generation of waste, recycling and the emission of toxic substances, knowing that such contamination can make us seriously ill and when this happens there is no reverse.

This is demonstrated by the data of the European Environment Agency in 2013, where there are about 30,000 deaths from exposure to nitrogen dioxide, small particles suspended in the air and ozone. Certain neurological diseases, metabolic disorders and some types of cancers, as you will see later in this book, are produced in the body by environmental agents, even more than by genetic conditions or unhealthy attitudes in the patient.

But, we are not the only ones affected. In fact, the entire animal kingdom suffers from pollution. In the last 69 years, not insignificant alterations have been discovered in various species across the planet. In Lake Michigan, United States, eagles and minks seem to have lost the instinct to mate and raise newborns, while the gulls of Lake Ontario and some alligators of Lake Apopka do not even know the light of the day they die before leaving the egg.

In Europe species simply disappear. Otters in some rivers in England, for example, and North Sea seals die massively every year.

It is not easy to find a relationship between human cancer, the loss of instinct in the eagles and the massive death of the seals, but it does exist. After many years of research it was discovered that the damage in common lies in the endocrine system and that it is caused by exposure to synthetic chemicals. Some pollutants and chemicals that are currently used in industry, have the ability to alter the hormonal system of any living being, are known as hormonal disruptors or endocrine disruptors, or by its acronym in English EDC (Endocrine disruptors).

In the next chapters we will examine in detail different types of EDCs and towards the end of the book we will list how to avoid exposure to this substance, a task that is not simple if one takes into account that the industry still uses them in the creation of many everyday objects.

For now, we will focus on elementary concepts to understand the urgency of these hormonal toxins.

What are endocrine disruptors?

An endocrine disruptor is a chemical with the ability to alter the hormonal system of the body. Its effect is to mimic or alter the effect of hormones, which causes confusing messages in the body and produces dysfunctions. These substances are minimally found in the natural state, usually from the industry and once in the body of any human or animal affects vital functions related to sexual growth and development.

The effect of endocrine disruptors is associated with various types of cancer, congenital malformations of the reproductive system, infertility, diabetes, precocious puberty, prostate conditions, behavioral disorders, loss of seminal quality, attention deficit, Parkinson's disease and disorders. cardiovascular, among other ailments.

The big problem with these substances and the reason why it is difficult to control them, is that their effect is cumulative and irreversible and can be transmitted from one generation to another even if the first one has not manifested any disease. We still don't know how EDCs can be eliminated, as Dr. Marisa López-Teijón, director of the Marqués Institute in Barcelona, states:

"All these substances remain inside the body accumulated because they cannot be degraded, just like when we see a plastic bag in the middle of the sea water. Keep swimming but there is no chance that nature knows how to eliminate it. "

Indeed, EDCs that come from pollution curiously act as contaminants in our body, but instead of floating in water they accumulate in adipose tissue and other organs for a long time. Since they became the object of study, these substances have been found in urine, breast milk (animal and human), blood, hair and amniotic fluid.

How are these substances classified?

There are many ways to classify endocrine disruptors, however, here we will only mention two to make understanding the subject a bit easier. According to their activity within the body, EDCs are classified as:

- **Estrogenomimetics:** Whose action is to bind to estrogenic receptors and mimic their natural action.

- **Antiandrogens:** They bind to estrogen receptors but do not activate them, that is, they antagonize their natural action.

They can also be classified according to their origin as:

- **Synthetics:** Whose origin is anthropological and linked to the industry.

- **Natural chemicals:** found in food for humans and animals.

Forms of exposure and dispersion through the environment

Contact with hormonal disruptors can occur through different pathways, for example, transfers from the mother to the fetus, breastfeeding, consumption of contaminated food and water, inhalation and absorption through the skin.
To recognize them more easily, it is convenient to generalize in the most potent forms of exposure, so you may come into contact with these substances by:

1.- Articles of daily use: Body creams, sun blockers, dentifrices, detergents and cleaning articles in general contain certain amounts of phthalates, brominated flame retardants and chlorinated paraffins, as they are used during their manufacture or storage.

These hormonal disruptors remain in the product but due to the use and exposure of the environment certain components migrate to water, soil or skin. For this reason babies and young children, whose tendency is to put objects in their mouths, are more likely to become contaminated, in fact, it is a great cause for alarm because it is known that many toys currently need various EDCs for their plasticization.

2.- Food: Food is one of the main sources of exposure to endocrine disruptors. The most risky foods of course are those that in their formation and growth are more exposed to herbicides, pesticides and emissions of the industry type, for example, fish and shellfish.

Natural fats such as oils and dairy products are also prone to accumulate high concentrations of EDC due to the affinity of these substances for lipids.

3.- Industry: The working hours in the industrial sector represent a risk of contamination with these substances since they are the place where they are generated. The most frequent current problems regarding this fact are male infertility and prostate cancer.

Likewise, some health disorders in childhood reflect a link with the parents' occupation and their contact with hormonal disruptors.

4.- Environment: Upon contact with air, water and soil contaminated with substances from industrial and agricultural activities. In this aspect, both rural environments, where there is livestock exploitation or crops, such as large cities, are affected in almost the same proportions.

Action mechanisms

It could be said that hormonal disruptors act as fakers in the body since once they have been incorporated they act on hormonal receptors and as their structure is similar to natural hormones, natural receptors bind and alter their normal functioning in three different ways .

One of the three possibilities with EDCs is that they block the union of natural hormones by taking their place, in this way no signal is sent and therefore no response is emitted. It acts as a mechanism of inhibition. The second possibility is to mimic, that is, copy the action of hormones, emit a signal and generate a response from it.

Finally there is the possibility of altering the normal concentrations of the hormone. In this case the receptors receive a signal that indicates that there is a level of hormone in the body and in response modifies the production, transport and excretion.

Once in the body, hormonal disruptors act in the manner described above, however, many factors influence their behavior in an individual. Let's examine some key points:

- **Action at very low doses:** Disruptors, like hormones, can act at very low concentrations, which is unfavorable because it is precisely the magnitude to which we are currently exposed.

- **Cocktail effect:** The vast majority of EDCs can act alone in the body or when mixed with other substances, as well as they can be activated, inhibited or diminished in the presence of other substances.

- **Biomagnification:** This type of substance is bioaccumulative, which means that they accumulate gradually in the organism of living beings, and it is transmitted from one organism to another as it advances through the trophic chain.

- **Exposure in moments of vulnerability:** Certain periods of life such as pregnancy and early childhood make the person more prone to contamination and damage caused by disruptors.

- **Substance in a state of latency:** Sometimes it can take years and decades before an illness caused by EDCs is manifested. Similarly, a generational jump can occur.

With this elementary information on endocrine disruptors we can dig a little deeper to know the most common hormonal toxins.

Part II The most common hormonal toxins

Chapter 2. Polychlorinated Biphenyl - PCBs

Polychlorinated biphenyl, better known as PCB, was first synthesized more than a century ago, approximately in 1881, at which time it was discovered that this substance is fire resistant, very stable, does not conduct electricity and is not very volatile at room temperature.

All these characteristics made the PCB the perfect candidate for the industry, but not for human contact. It was not until several years later that the effects on health began to be noticed.

The polychlorinated biphenyl is basically formed by chlorine, carbon and hydrogen and at the molecular level its structure forms two rings, so it is extremely stable and resistant to chemical and biological rupture through natural processes, in other words, living organisms and Natural cycles cannot metabolize it.

PCBs in everyday life

The ban on the use of PCBs took place in 1972, the United States being the first country to establish the standard and eventually other nations, however, the effects of the substance are still present.

According to a study on veterinary toxicology carried out by Bursian S. in 2012, about 31% of the total PCB produced years ago is maintained in the global ecosystem and more than 780 thousand tons are kept in old abandoned electrical equipment in the field or Stored without efficient controls.

Similarly, biphenyls are present in dielectric fluids, heat exchangers and capacitors, but also in pesticide diluents, welds, adhesives, tracing papers, metal carving and turbine lubricants.

Contamination risk

If the PCBs stopped being used almost forty years ago and are mainly found in turbines and old equipment, they do not seem a close threat, however, contamination with this substance is not as complicated as it seems, only specific situations must occur for this to occur.

When a transformer breaks down, due to vandalism, accidents, negligence or explosions, the biphenyl enters the environment and expands through rainwater and runoff that eventually comes into contact with the ground and enters the trophic chain where it will pass from a living being to other.

As it is a very low biodegradable substance, it has been considered a Persistent Organic Pollutant (COP), this means that it remains in the environment for long periods, which even cover centuries.

Chapter 3. Polychlorinated Dioxins

"Dioxins" is the generic term used to designate a very large group of COP compounds. It is estimated that there are about 75 substances of this type and all of them have in common the element chlorine in their molecular structure.

DDPCs, as dioxins are normally known, are not synthesized in laboratories or in any industry sector, in fact they come from other chemical substances that are exposed to combustion and although it could be considered a relief, in reality, it is an even more powerful trigger.

Where do dioxins come from?

In the paper industry, during the classic bleaching process molecular chlorine or hypochlorite is used, which also contains chlorine, and both substances when reacting with the carbon structures present in the wood give rise to the dioxins that eventually pass into the environment.

Another way in which these substances are born is through various manufacturing processes involving chlorinated substances, such as chlorophenols, which are used as antiseptics, herbicides, preservatives, disinfectants, pesticides and wood preservatives.

DDPCs are also released into the air and the atmosphere in general, through emissions from solid waste incinerators, through the gases emitted by everyday vehicles, cigarette smoke and oil plants. The numerous sources of this substance at the urban level are very alarming, in our daily lives.
Finally, they are one of the few endocrine disruptors that can be achieved in nature. They form during volcanic activity or

forest fires and their pure state is clearly crystalline, but when mixed with ashes and other compounds it loses that appearance.

How dangerous are they?

We could say that a dioxin is dangerous depending on the type of substance it is. As we said before, there are hundreds of dioxins but the most toxic one is 2,3,7,8-TCDD or 2,3,7,8-tetrachlorodibenzo-p-dioxin.

The International Agency for Research on Cancer (IARC) and the Department of Health of the United States consider tetrachlorodibenzo a potential carcinogen and a very dangerous substance in general.

TCDD is responsible for various metabolic, neuromuscular and central nervous system effects. It is also known to have teratogenic effects, that is, it is an agent capable of causing a congenital defect or mutation in the embryo during pregnancy.

Chlorocné is one of the best known effects of TCDD, it consists of a rash similar to adolescent acne, but pimples and cysts are produced by the disappearance of the sebaceous glands due to exposure to this substance. One of the biggest risks of this substance is its ability to disperse. The larger particles, due to their weight, will be deposited near their source, that is, the soil or water near the incinerator or factory, but the rest evaporates and is transported in any direction.

Once in the water or on the earth, dioxins easily enter the food chain and it is a matter of time before they reach our body.

Chapter 4. Organochlorine pesticides

A pesticide is a substance that eradicates certain animals and plants, which for the purpose of a crop are considered pests. Nature does not resort to these types of practices because the order that governs ecosystems is responsible for the regulation of each species, but since the natural system has been broken, we humans must resort to chemical weapons designed by ourselves.

Organochlorine compounds are substances that were widely used in the last century to create pesticides, at that time dichlorodiphenyltrichloroethane (DDT) was the preferred compound, it was even used to control the Anopheles mosquito, which transmits malaria.

The big problem with DDT, and with the other organochlorine compounds of the "dirty dozen" is its high chemical stability. Their ring-shaped structure makes them great resources for exterminating pests, but once inside the animal organism it continues to cause damage.

The organochlorines to the sun today

The use of DDT for the manufacture of pesticides was banned in the United States approximately in 1972 and great efforts have been made to minimize the use of other organochlorines after the Stockholm Convention, however, these substances are still kept in the atmosphere since the date.

Many countries still use DDT and other substances in some household products to eliminate insects, so it is convenient to analyze the exposure factors that put us at risk.

Pollution of the atmosphere: For faster, pesticides are normally applied with sprayers, so it is very easy to contaminate the air in this way and allow the transport of the substance to other regions or to rise to other levels of the atmosphere where they react to sunlight and the other compounds that are already there.

Soil: Organochlorine substances are incorporated into the soil by absorbing the substance after spraying or also by air. Once deposited here they pass to the bodies of water, or undergo degradation and evaporation processes.

Water bodies: Organochlorine pesticides and the substances that are produced when they come into contact with the environment are transported by air or soil to aquatic ecosystems, and from there several possibilities are born. These substances can biomagnify, degrade, remain unchanged or return to the atmosphere through the water cycle.

The ultimate goal of these routes is, of course, adipose tissue and certain plant foods, since they are water-insoluble substances but similar to lipids, as evidenced by a study carried out in Sweden in the 70s, where DDT was found in pigs and cattle.

Thus, this endocrine disruptor whose mission is to attack the pests of our food does not stop fulfilling its work once it reaches our body and although it does not affect us in the same way, it certainly generates damage to our health.

THE DIRTY DOCENA

There are twelve substances used worldwide, which due to their chemical nature became a great conflict. Within the group we find:

Pesticides: Aldrin, Chlordane, Dieldrin, Endrin, Heptachlor, Mirex, Toxaphene and DDT.

Industrial products: Hexachlorobenzene and Polychlorobiphenyls.

Waste from industrial activity: Dioxins and Furans.

Chapter 5. Perfluorinated substances

The fifth endocrine disruptor that we will present in the book is not traveling in the atmosphere or in the water as it happens with the previous ones, it entered your house at the time that you bought certain things of daily use.

Non-stick pans, special carpet cleaning detergents, certain waterproof garments, lubricants, floor polishes and some hair products contain perfluorinated substances, as do certain pesticides and emulsions used on an industrial level.

The family of perfluorinated compounds is numerous but the most toxic ones are perfluorooctane sulphonate (PFOS) and perfluorooctanoate (PFOA), which according to the Stockholm Convention classify as Persistent Organic Pollutants (POPs).

Once the risk of perfluorinated substances was discovered, measures were taken to avoid their use, one of them was replacing the most dangerous ones with others of the same family that were not a threat, but according to the experts' opinion this is not enough.

In a number of the magazine Environmental Health Perspectives, of the year 2015, the "Declaration of Madrid" was published, a call for attention by more than 200 scientists who claim that the manufacturers of perfluorinated substances do not offer enough information about their toxicity and that in addition, alternatives without fluoride should be sought, since that would be a definitive solution.

Using perfluorinated substances of the same family cannot be a true solution since degradation can cause PFOS or PFOA, or generate their own toxicological effects.

PFC, pregnancy and lactation

As perfluorinated substances are in our own home, pregnancy and young children are the most susceptible due to their natural condition, in fact, they are the main affected. According to a study on perfluorinated immunotoxicity, conducted by Philippe Grandjean of the University of Southern Denmark, PFC's can generate testicular cancer in children exposed during pregnancy or affect their immune system.

In another study carried out by Damià Barceló, director of the Catalan Institute for Water Research (ICRA), the breast milk of twenty women with newborn children was analyzed and in 99% of the cases, low numbers of PFCs were found, however , a single woman showed a high level, which turned the food into a risk for the infant, as recommended by the European Food Safety Authority

On the other hand, when analyzing infant formulas and cereal foods for babies, Damià Barceló discovered PFCs in low doses and it is assumed that they come from packaging and thus demonstrated two important things: (1) First, the vast majority of the population has a certain amount of perfluorinated substances in their body; and (2) in second, we must be very careful when caring for a newborn baby or child.

Chapter 6. Phthalates

Phthalates are a family of substance composed in total, by eighty synthetically created members. In the industry its price is very low and it turns out to be a very versatile material, so it has been used extensively since its creation.

Currently, you can get these substances in paints and varnishes, toys, modeling clays, cosmetics, building materials, cleaning products, medical supplies, adhesives and household adhesives, printer inks, fabrics and pesticides.

Phthalates are mainly used as plasticizers, they are incorporated into vinyl, for example, to soften it and make it flexible and resistant. It is also used as a scent fixer, as is the case with cleaning products and cosmetics. Previously, it was widely used to make toys and baby items, but thanks to the ease with which the compound migrates and lodges in the body, its use was prohibited.

How do they get to us?

Phthalates do not chemically bind to the other substances with which they are mixed, so they gradually release as time goes by, are used or exposed to heat. Thus, exposure to these substances is continuous and cumulative. Think of all the plastic things you are exposed to every day and for how long.

In addition to this, phthalates are emitted by any industry that uses the substance at any stage of its manufacturing process, so that there is no escape, they are present in the entire population but to a greater or lesser extent, however, their action does not It is immediate, it may be years before the manifestation of any symptoms.

Luis Domínguez, professor of toxicology at the Faculty of Medicine of the Las Palmas University of Gran Canaria, explains that phthalates enter through the skin, through the respiratory or digestive tract, pass into the bloodstream and are distributed throughout the body and they reach the tissue cells, where they wait indefinitely.

Hopefully, prohibitive measures have been established around these substances, but this has not yielded the expected results. An investigation carried out in the American population indicates that in the organism of the 11,000 people studied, phthalates, whose use is prohibited, were replaced by new ones not yet regulated.

It seems then that we live very close to these substances, we could consider them a chemical element as usual for us as oxygen, but how harmful it could be for our health and what measures we can take, remains to be seen.

Chapter 7. Bisphenol-A

The seventh endocrine disruptor on the list, is very associated with food, in fact, when eating a packaged food there is a great possibility that you are taking a certain dose of bisphenol-A to your body.

Bisphenol-A or BPA, is an industrial chemical that has been used as a coating for tin cans for more than fifty years and to manufacture polycarbonate plastics, resins and CDs.

Water bottles, plastic food containers, baby bottles, certain toys for infants and soda containers are some everyday products that expose us to this substance. As you can see, bisphenol is common for us given the constant use of plastic.

According to the Center for Disease Control and Prevention (CDC) more than 90% of Americans have traces of BPA in the body, however, not exceeding the "tolerable daily dose." Children, on the other hand, do not run so lucky. The European Food Safety Authority (AESA), in 2013, published a report explaining that children aged 3 to 10 are much more exposed to bisphenol because food consumption, regarding their body weight, It is superior during that period than in other ages.

From packaging to the body

BPA, like many other endocrine disruptors, is present in the air, water and soil, but in small quantities that do not represent a very large risk, the problem actually arises when this chemical is released from the plastic that contains it and passes to food.

BPA migration can occur from a bottle to the liquid, at the time a container is heated in the microwave, when it is frozen or when it is kept inside the refrigerator. With "safe plastics" this tries to minimize.

Polyethylene Terephthalate (PET) and Polypropylene (PP) are two materials that transmit up to 0.01 mg / kg, a lower amount compared to cans and other types of plastics that are used for the same purpose.

Bisphenol-A Migration

In order for Bisphenol to leave the plastic certain specific conditions must occur, for example, when the pH of the food is low (acidic) the migration is higher, such is the case of citrus juices, tomato sauce and carbonated drinks.

In the same way, the deterioration of the plastic, the temperature, the exposure time and the type of material used to make the container influence the amount of bisphenol that passes into the food.

Chapter 8. Parabens

If we continue to take a tour of the house in search of endocrine disruptors that have infiltrated, the next place we should check is the bathroom, here you will get parabens, one of the most used chemicals in the cosmetic industry.

Parabens are chemicals that are used as preservatives in products beauty products and certain drugs. The reason why it is used is that with it a bactericidal and fungicidal effect is obtained, that is, it prevents the growth of microorganisms in the product, in addition, it is economical.

80% of cosmetics on the market contain parabens, and approximately 90% of them are synthetic. Organic parabens, typical of some plants and fruits, are metabolized in the body and do not represent a problem, for example, blueberries.

On the labels of certain products you can see the names of the different members of the paraben family, usually in English, such as methylparaben, propylparaben, butylparaben and benzylparaben. Also some other industrial products contain these substances.

Fish cans, milk-based preparations, jams, oils, strains, nasal and eye drops and shaving foams also contain parabens and basically fulfill the same function: prevent the proliferation of bacteria and extend the shelf life of the product.

They're safe?

For more than fifteen years it was thought that parabens are substances of low toxicity and very safe since the body absorbs, metabolizes and expels them, so no restrictions were created regarding their use, however, years later that idea It was replaced by a not very encouraging one.

In 2004, a group of oncologists from the University of Reading, Edinburgh, studied carcinogenic tissues and 90% of the samples from breast cancer patients were contaminated with traces of parabens. According to the Cosmetic Ingredient Review (CIR) studies, the use of parabens in cosmetics is not a risk in amounts below 25% and the concentration of the substance usually varies between 0.01 to 0.3%.

The opinion of many scientists and doctors diverges regarding the effects of this substance on health, but many agree that they are causing allergies. Contact dermatitis, inflammation, redness and dry skin are symptoms of a reaction to parabens when the skin or scalp is exposed to cosmetics, dyes, creams and some medications.

Chapter 9. Triclosan

In the bathroom next to the parabens is triclosan, the ninth disruptor on the list and one of the most related to hygiene, especially the mouth and teeth.

Triclosan is a chemical compound that, like parabens, is used as a preservative because it inhibits the growth of bacterial colonies. It is currently in more than two thousand products in the market and as expected, it is also within our agency.

In a study carried out in the United States, triclosan was found in about 75% of the urine samples analyzed, in people of different ages and of both genders and of course, its presence in the organism generates effects on health. This leads us to question why this substance is used so much.

Triclosan is present in dentifrices, mouthwashes, deodorants, shower gels, makeup and nail cleaning products, it is also used at the pharmaceutical level, but its increase in the market actually took place when toothpastes were created "Total protection".

When discovering the great bactericidal effect, the industry thought that oral hygiene products with this chemical would solve gingivitis and bad breath, which originate in the proliferation of bacteria and although, it was a wise decision in that aspect it was not taken considering the negative effect it generates.

According to the European Union, the maximum allowed concentration that does not compromise health is 0.3% for toothpastes and body soaps; In mouthwash it is up to 0.2%, however, this does not consider the cumulative effect it can have on toothbrushes.

The same study conducted by chemists at the University of Massachusetts Amherst revealed that the accumulation of triclosan in toothbrush bristles can be raised seven to twelve times above the recommended daily exposure dose.

Triclosan in the environment

Triclosan not only stays in the bathroom of your house, it is also present in the environment. In general, the substance reaches aquatic environments - both rivers and sea - through sewage, but it can also pass to other ecosystems through discarded toothbrushes and industrial production wastes.

The effect of triclosan when it is in the environment is resistance. Its natural function as a chemical is to respond as a bactericide and that does in the first instance, but after a period of time the surviving microorganisms become stronger creating resistance.

For this reason, the Food and Drug Administration (FDA) suggests its complete withdrawal from the market. When an organism creates resistance to a substance it becomes immune to it, so treating an infection, for example, will be more complicated.

Chapter 10. Musks

If we continue to analyze the cosmetics present in your bathroom, in addition to triclosan and parabens we would find musks, coming from long-lasting body perfumes, whose shelf life is so long that scientists have obtained samples of perfumes in lakes and rivers.

A musk is considered to be a fatty substance with a strong odor, secreted by the deer and musk ox glands, in addition to other animals and plants with a similar odor. Previously, these chemicals were obtained from the death of the animal and the extraction of the oil from the plant, but the industry soon took care of replicating it synthetically to obtain them in a larger volume.

In this way, today we get polycyclic musks, galaxolide, and tonalide and two types of nitrogen musks, all of them main ingredients in the manufacture of perfumes.

Synthetic musks do not break down in the environment, as with natural musks, they remain intact for decades, even when they have already lodged in the adipose tissue of some animal or human, where they can cause disease.

According to the journal Environmental Science and Technology, musks have been found in human fatty tissue and in breast milk and it is not yet known what the effects are, however, some animal studies indicate that these substances might be responsible for alterations in the endocrine system and certain types of cancer.

An unnecessary exposure

If the function of perfumes is analyzed compared to that of other cosmetics, it could be concluded that it is a dispensable product, because our hygiene and health does not depend on it, on the contrary, it exposes us and compromises the environment around us.

Synthetic musks, like many other substances, are integrated into the food chain and pass from one spice to another with unfortunate effects or remain in the ecosystem for years, polluting at different levels, as is the case with our body.

Samples of synthetic musks have been found in blood, fat, human milk, and even in newborn children, who receive them from their mothers throughout pregnancy.

It seems that of all endocrine disruptors studied so far, synthetic musks pay a very high price for the product obtained, which does not appear as a necessity, since its implementation in perfumes affects from the bodies of water to the body of newborns.

Chapter 11. Ultraviolet filters

Sun creams are one of the most recommended products for the protection and care of the skin because they have the surprising ability to act as an invisible armor against the powerful rays of the sun, but while they are healthy for our skin, the rest of our body It does not benefit in the same way.

In almost any sunscreen on the market we will get avobenzone, oxybenzone, ecamsule and octocrylene, chemicals that the Food and Drug Administration (FDA) considered safe until recently. This health agency carried out this year 2019 an investigation published in the journal JAMA, in which it was discovered that the four compounds named above are absorbed through the skin and directed to the bloodstream, where they remain more than 24 hours after application and accumulate with daily exposure to the substance.

To reach these conclusions, four commercial presentations of sunscreens were used among 24 people (12 men and 12 women) and the participants were asked to apply the product four times a day for four days, after this time the concentrations were analyzed in blood.

The results reflect that avobenzone, oxybenzone, ecamsule and octocrylene exceed the recommended index only on the first day of use and that in addition, oxybenzone can reach even seven days of permanence, being able to stay in breast milk.

The FDA believes that while the four chemicals exceed the recommended daily limit are not a health threat, however, research is still needed to prove their true effect on plasma concentrations.

Damage to the marine ecosystem

It has been shown that oxybenzone, which is found in approximately 60% of sunscreens in any of its presentations, is responsible for significant damage to marine ecosystems, especially coral reefs.

In a study published in the Archives of Environmental Contamination and Toxicology, researchers diluted oxybenzone in different concentrations in tanks with coral larvae and after eight hours of exposure they lost mobility, coloration and adopted an atypical circular shape

.

The effect of the highest concentrations was the most surprising since they caused DNA lesions and therefore the death of corals. The study was repeated in different areas and in all cases the same effects were observed.

In humans, the effect is not as drastic as in corals, however, we must take into account that studies have yet to be carried out to deepen the effect of the substance on the organism.

Chapter 12. Organophosphorus pesticides

The twelfth disruptor that will be announced in this book is widely used in the fields, where the fruits and vegetables that we bring to our table grow every day. Unfortunately the people most exposed to it are agricultural workers, however, the substance can easily reach the cities, where we live.

Organophosphorus pesticides, very common in large crops, are made from organic compounds that in their structure have several phosphorus atoms and act as inhibitors of certain enzymes responsible for the functioning of the nervous system. The toxic effect of phosphorus compounds is well known and despite this, numerous accidents occur every year. In Central America alone, it is estimated that 3% of agricultural workers exposed to pesticides suffer acute poisoning every year.

Organophosphorus compounds, such as chlorpyriflora (CPF) for example, at high and very high doses produce neurotoxic effects, but it was unknown what happened with low concentrations until a group of Argentine scientists dedicated themselves to discover it and surprised the health authorities with the results.

Small dose damage

Researchers from the Faculties of Pharmacy and Biochemistry and Medicine of the University of Buenos Aires, and scientists from the National University of Comahue, studied the effects of exposure to low doses of chlorpyrifos in rats and cell cultures. Both objects of study were analyzed separately.

The amount of chlorpyrifos to which the experimental animals were exposed was the daily intake admitted and the maximum dose in which no effects were observed. When female rats were observed, these presented changes in breast tissue and hyperplasia and the researchers discovered active cell proliferation and migration pathways.

In male rats the effect showed that chlorpyrifos acts as an endocrine disruptor. The test animals were neutered and did not have the possibility of producing hormones, however, the presence of the substance generated an inhibition of the pituitary hypothalamus axis, that is, it acted as if it were an endogenous estrogen.

On the other hand, the cell lines received selected doses below where 50% of the cells die and different behaviors were observed in the estrogen-dependent and independent cells, both models being breast carcinogenesis.

Dependent cells when exposed to low doses of CPF induced cell proliferation and increased the effect of migration, a classic mechanism of tumor progression. In estrogen independent cell lines, only death due to chemical imbalance plus non-proliferation or migration occurred.

The conclusions of this extensive study are alarming because this chemical compound is used very widely, so the public health problem that could be generated from it would have proportions equally large to those of its use.

Chapter 13. Tributyltin

In order to know this new disruptor, we must locate ourselves in the marine coasts, more specifically in the vessels, which are the main source of emission of tributyltin, one of the most dangerous substances for aquatic life.

The external walls of the boats and turbines are covered with a special paint based on tributyltin or TBT, thus avoiding encrustation or biofouling, which is the colonization of the structure by marine organisms. When mollusks, algae and bacteria take over the surface of a vessel, it makes it slower and therefore, there is greater fuel consumption, in addition to the fact that in the vast majority of cases, very expensive damages occur in the metal.

To avoid all these discomforts in the early sixties, anti-fouling paints containing arsenic, mercury and different pesticides were used, but it was expensive and eventually the tributyltin was considered a much more profitable solution, however, the price that pays for life Marina is quite high.

More than just a repellent

The original idea of the antifouling paints was to keep the problematic species away from the surface of the boats, but resulted in excessive damage due to the chemical nature of the compound.

Tributyltin (TBT) has a tin atom and three butyl groups, so it has very little water solubility, in fact, the compound prefers to bind to the suspended particles and sediments of the seabed, once here it begins to generate problems in aquatic organisms. It has been shown that TBT is responsible for deformation in oyster shells, neurotoxic and teratogenic effects, that is, embryo mutations. In addition, it generates an effect called "imposex", which consists in the imposition of sex changes in gastropods (snails).

According to a research carried out in 2017 by Norma Sbarbati, in Argentina, TBT in mollusks can cause sterility and increased mortality and cause DNA damage, but they are not the only species, mammals are also affected by Similarly.

The decrease in spermatogenesis, obesity, malformations and lymphocyte inhibition, were some of the effects observed in different laboratory studies involving mice and it is not difficult to expose a mammal to this substance, since it is not only used in ships, but also It is used in wood treatment, textile cleaning and PVC manufacturing.

Chapter 14. Solvents and aliphenols

The alkylphenols are a group of chemical substances that are used industrially to manufacture surfactants, a product with the ability to reduce the surface hardness of water.

The aliphenols cause the molecules to slip together and cannot adhere, so they inevitably interact with the oil and fat in the environment. Knowing this it is very easy to guess where this substance is found: in detergents, soaps, foaming agents and emulsifiers.

It is estimated that the annual production of alkylphenols is close to 500,000 tons worldwide and that approximately 60% of them are discharged into the aquatic environment after use. Likewise, 80% corresponds to octylphenol and nonylphenol, the two most used but most toxic alkylphenols.

Our clothes are contaminated

Alkylphenols are present in textile finishing products, as evidenced by research conducted by Greenpeace in 2003 in which household dust was studied and the presence of phthalates, organostannic compounds, formaldehyde and alkylphenols was detected.

These substances are used to stamp, prevent wear on the fabric and confer certain cleaning properties, but their permanence in the tissue is ephemeral and the particles are slowly released into the environment.

In that year Greenpeace analyzed the garments of the most important companies and found the presence of ethoxylated nonylphenol in more than fourteen brands. The most alarming thing according to the organization is that nonylphenol is a very potent endocrine disruptor.

Another way to contaminate our garments and expose ourselves to alkylphenols is through the constant use of laundry detergents and soaps, which has the extra to contaminate water and as a consequence, marine environments, lakes and rivers.

Sexual development and alkylphenols

Several experiments carried out in recent years show that rodents exposed to nonylphenol, before and after birth, develop smaller testicles and less sperm at maturity, even if it is a small amount of the substance.

Fish also have an affected sexual development, but they appear hermaphroditism. Investigations carried out in some bodies of water in the United Kingdom indicated that fish with this problem were concentrated right at the discharge points of the purification and purification plants of domestic waters.

Clothing is our second skin and for scientists it is disturbing that such a harmful substance is so close to us. It remains to be seen how science addresses this situation so compromising for our health.

Chapter 15. Styrene

The fifteenth endocrine disruptor on the list is one of the few that our body is able to assimilate and discard a few hours after being contaminated, however, we are so exposed to styrene and the human body is so sensitive to its absorption that it can result As dangerous as the rest.

Styrene is a liquid substance that is produced both in nature and in industry, certain microorganisms such as bacteria and fungi produce styrene in their metabolic processes. For us, the substance is a threat when it comes from combustion and manufacturing processes.

Packaging materials, carpets, glass fibers and insulators contain styrene in the form of long chains known as polystyrene and at the industrial level large amounts of the substance are released during the manufacture of all these elements.

Styrene in our body

Thanks to industrial activity, styrene is present in the air, soil and water in almost every city in the world and to a lesser extent in rural environments. In soil and water it can be degraded by the action of microorganisms or evaporate into the atmosphere, in the air its degradation deserves a couple of days.

Styrene enters our body through inhalation, ingestion or contact with the substance, it is enough to touch with our fingers some product that contains it so that it enters directly through the dermis.

The same happens when food acquires the substance thanks to the packaging, but in this case they come to us through ingestion. We inhale styrene from the environment and those who are most exposed are factory workers.

Once in our body, 85% of styrene is removed in 24 hours through urine and approximately 5% through the air we exhale, but this short period is enough to cause damage to the body.

Rats exposed to high doses of styrene suffer from alterations in the learning process and damage of sperm in adulthood, in addition The National Toxicology Program of the US Department of Health and Human Services classifies styrene as "reasonably anticipated to be a carcinogen "

Remember that the effect that a substance can have on the organism depends on exposure time and its concentration, so it is not surprising that styrene leaves traces on our body even when it is not stored in the tissue.

Chapter 16. Chlorinated paraffins

Chlorinated paraffins or PCCC are one of the most invasive chemical substances in the industry and, in turn, one with the greatest dispersal capacity, so much so that small percentages of this chemical have been found in various Arctic species, which are presumed to be very remote and Away from the big cities.

PCCCs are water insoluble liquids with great chemical stability and are released into the atmosphere during their production, storage, transport and use, in other words, they are released into the environment and basically contaminate throughout their life cycle.

Paraffins are used in the manufacture of plastics, paints and industrial lubricants, but chlorinated paraffins have also been found in toys, stickers, textiles, sports equipment and kitchen utensils at a concentration of 11%, which exceeds the levels allowed by health agencies

PCCC has been detected in the air, water from rivers and lakes, sewage, fish, mammals and remote regions such as the Arctic, this is because in environmental conditions the substance degrades very slowly but thanks to industrial production They accumulate very fast.

Paraffins enter the food chain through aquatic organisms, they are the first to expose themselves and mammals become contaminated by feeding on them. This explains why PCCC has been measured in the breast milk of Inuit women in Northern Quebec and in the indigenous tribes of North America.

Dangerous for the Stockholm Convention

In 2017, the chlorinated paraffins were included in Annex A of the agreement in the Stockholm Convention, which means that the substance must be eliminated and also its mixing with other types of compounds is limited. To date, paraffins had not been deeply studied as a threat to human health.

In a two-year study carried out by the United States National Toxicology Program, the effect of exposure of female and male mice to chlorinated paraffins was evaluated. The changes observed in the mice were changes in breathing, decreased activity, spinal problems, adenomas and hepatocellular carcinomas.

Such a study concluded that it was necessary to verify the effects that they could have on humans and soon the International Agency for Research on Cancer considered that some PCCCs are possible carcinogens.

Chapter 17. Lead

Until this chapter we have listed various chemical substances that act as endocrine disruptors, most of them are synthesized and then incorporated into industrial processes, but this does not happen with lead and the next metals to mention, they already exist in nature but their use in our activities makes them a danger.

Lead is a toxic metal found in the earth's crust, it was discovered in 1899 and its possible applications were quickly studied. Today the damage that lead causes in human health is known to everyone, however, the substance is already present everywhere.

Where is the lead?

This metal is used to make some cosmetics, toys, medicines, enamels, jewelry, paints, fuels and is used in the metalworking industry for welding. In the same way it is obtained through mining and through recycling.

Lead emissions reach water, air and land and at this point the contamination of species, including humans, continues. A common way in which we expose ourselves to lead is through drinking water channeled through pipes made of lead or welded with this metal.

What does lead do in our body?

Lead enters the body through intestinal absorption, through the skin and by inhalation and once inside it is transported in the bloodstream to all organs and tissues, usually accumulates in the bones, teeth, livers, brain , spleen, kidneys and lungs. During pregnancy it crosses the placenta.

The vapor containing lead allows 50% absorption by the body, which quickly affects the soft organs and prevents the fixation of iron in the blood, causing anemia.

One of the best known conditions caused by lead is called "saturnism" and is a form of poisoning that blocks the synthesis of hemoglobin and alters the transport of oxygen to the blood.

Lead and reproductive development

Mothers exposed to this metal show a high rate of abortions and stillbirths, babies with low birth weight and premature births also have a higher incidence. Several studies show that men's fertility decreases when the blood lead level exceeds 40ug / dl or is maintained at 25ug / dl for several years. Metal affects the spermatogenesis process and generates menstrual disorders in women.

In adolescents, the effect it causes is the delay of sexual maturation according to a study by the National Health and Nutrition Examination Survey conducted in the United States.

Menarche, the appearance of pubic hair and breast development are significantly delayed when the blood lead concentration exceeds 40ug / dl.

These are just some of the effects that lead has on health. We are facing one of the most toxic metals, which compromises especially the health of children, whose body weight and habits make them more vulnerable.

Chapter 18. Cadmium

Cadmium is a natural metal that has the curious property of acting as a true endocrine disruptor, once it enters the body it competes with estrogen receptors and sends erratic signals to the body. No doubt this is one of its most dangerous effects.

This heavy metal is not free, it is usually associated with zinc, lead and copper and is obtained by smelting and refining, only cadmium is found purely through the greenockite which is a metal sulfide .

Volcanic activity, rock erosion and forest fires release certain amounts of cadmium into the atmosphere, but the greatest emission comes from human industrial activity.

How does cadmium get to us?

Cadmium reaches our body through ingestion and inhalation, as do other synthetic disruptors. The application of chemical fertilizers adds to the soil and water this metal and plants and animals create some resistance to it, but transmit it to us when we feed on them.

Fish and mollusks, which are contaminated by water and plankton intake have high concentrations of cadmium in their tissues, as do mussels, algae and some fungi such as mushrooms.

Cocoa and tobacco also incorporate cadmium into their biomass. When a person smokes, it generates cadmium oxide that is absorbed by the body quickly and it is estimated that 50% of all the metal that is inhaled in this way enters the bloodstream.

Cadmium as an endocrine disruptor

Cadmium is able to bind and activate the estrogen receptor □, in fact, it competes with natural estrogen to take its place in our body and when it succeeds it induces cell proliferation and increases the expression of genes regulated by this hormone.

One of the probable effects is the early arrival of puberty, the weight gain of the uterus and the development of the glands in young women, in men it is possible to decrease semen quality and alterations in sex hormones.

On the other hand, pregnant women exposed to cadmium may experience spontaneous abortions and fetuses contaminated under birth weight. It has also been shown that cadmium decreases the synthesis of leptin, a hormone that regulates organogenesis and fetal development.
.

Knowing that cadmium is one of the most used metals in the industry should be one of our priorities to find ways to protect ourselves, but that will be discussed later in this book.

Chapter 19. Nickel

The metal that follows in our list of powerful endocrine disruptors is nickel, whose solid appearance is white-silver and is used to make stainless steel, coins, jewels, valves and heat exchangers.

Our contact with nickel is both direct and indirect, it reaches our body through food and water but also through kitchen utensils and jewelry and although the body does not absorb large amounts of metal through the skin approximately 20 % of the population is sensitive and experiences dermatitis, redness and itching.

Nickel in food

Nickel is released into the environment by natural and anthropogenic sources, for example through the combustion of coal and oil, the manufacture of alloys, electroplating and incineration of waste.

An important percentage of the metal is fixed in the soil by plants and is introduced into our body by ingesting its fruits. In acidic soils, nickel metal has even more mobility and therefore seeps into the deep layers until it reaches groundwater.

In some places like India, Gopi and Kumar, various studies have shown that the main source of nickel contamination in aquatic environments comes from ship debris and its anti-corrosive paints. In the Mediterranean, pollution of marine water bodies and therefore of the species that inhabit them comes from agriculture, industry and land development.

Once the mollusks and fish integrate nickel into their tissues they pass to us when they eat them and apparently the cooking process increases the concentration of the metal due to the loss of water.

If a food manages to reach our kitchen without being contaminated with nickel, it is very likely that it loses its purity when it comes into contact with the kitchen utensils and exposes itself to heat, since the metal is present in the stainless steel and the stone and is progressively released with the use.

Nickel and the endocrine system

The mammalian body's neuroendocrine system is particularly affected by nickel salts, which induce alterations in prolactin and luteinizing hormone levels, two hormones involved in female reproductive functions.

In a study conducted in 356 Russian women workers of a nickel refinery, an increase in the rate of spontaneous abortions (15.9%) was observed, compared to the rate corresponding to 342 local women with another occupation (8.5%).

On the other hand, in studies with rats and mice a testicular degeneration was observed when the animals were exposed to nickel sulfate. It is also known that this metal is genotoxic, which means that it produces some genetic abnormalities.

If the cell exhibits any abnormality and is unable to reverse the changes, the cell cycle continues with the error and this can lead to uncontrolled proliferation, alteration of cell apoptosis and finally to the development of cancer.

Given the risks suggested by exposure to nickel, it should become a concern for us to avoid contact with the metal and its more toxic forms, because although inhalation and intake is not absorbed quickly through the skin, it enters our body significant quantities.

Chapter 20. Mercury

Mercury is one of the most well-known toxic metals, in fact, prevention campaigns have been carried out in Spain and other European countries in which pregnant women are invited to avoid the consumption of fish, shellfish and shellfish during pregnancy.

Mercury is a very toxic silver white metal, the only one at 0 ° C is in a liquid state. This chemical element is not essential in any biological process, however, it accumulates very easily in most living things.

In nature you can find mercury in the form of sulphides of mercury, arsenic, iron and antimony, but it can also be linked to other minerals such as zinc, copper, gold and lead.

How does mercury reach our body?

Mercury can enter the respiratory, digestive or cutaneous route, the first being one of the most effective. Both elemental and inorganic mercury and its derivative compounds reach the blood with an efficiency of 80% after inhalation, that is, 80% of the inhaled substance reaches the bloodstream.

On the other hand, the gastrointestinal tract inorganic mercury is absorbed in 0.01% because the metal does not interact with other biomolecules, while inorganic mercury compounds are absorbed between 2 and 15%, depending on their solubility. Organic compounds by ingestion are absorbed by 95%.

The greatest emission of mercury to the environment comes from the metallurgical industry and from the wastewater of the cities, every year approximately one thousand tons of the metal are released from sewage networks to the earth's surface.

Effect of mercury in the body

Mercury has the ability to precipitate the proteins synthesized by cells, mainly from neurons and inhibits the sulfydryl groups of several essential enzymes, thus alters the metabolic and enzymatic systems, also inhibits the synthesis of proteins in the mitochondria and blocks their function energetic

As for the effect it can have on children, scientists have not reached conclusive evidence. In Spain, the INMA Project (Children and the Environment) was carried out, in which the concentration of mercury in 1800 newborns from Valencia, Sabadell, Asturias and Guipúzcoa was analyzed.

The levels in newborns were high with a rate of 24% higher as recommended by the World Health Organization and 64% above the recommendation of the United States Environmental Protection Agency.

The effects of mercury in children can vary from cognitive problems to premature delivery. There is no established toxicity limit for mercury, it is generally accepted between 50 and 160 µg / day, but given the extent of this chemical element it is necessary to make provisions in this regard.

Chapter 21. Arsenic

The last endocrine disruptor on the list is a potently carcinogenic metal with multiple effects both in the short and long term. Currently, various health organizations have set limits in industries to control exposure to the substance, however, it is difficult to manage once it has spread through the atmosphere.

Arsenic is a natural element present in the earth's crust, in the air, water and earth. This metal exists in different oxidation states and each one has higher or lower levels of toxicity.

Thus, exposure to arsenic is not difficult, it is mainly due to water and intake of contaminated products. Throughout the world the most contaminated foods are fish and shellfish, red and white meat, rice and seaweed.

How is arsenic found in food?

As arsenic can be found in various ways, it is associated with food and the environment in different ways, for example, in drinking water it is found inorganic form as arsenate and arsenite, in rice it is found inorganic form and in algae marine like arseno-sugars.
Some studies done to measure the efficiency of the metal in the body showed that in rodents the inorganic arsenic is absorbed in 95%, that is, almost in its entirety, while in rice plants in 89%, therefore when we consume these foods we expose ourselves significantly.

What effect does it have on the body?

Arsenic metal causes multiple alterations in numerous molecular, cellular and enzymatic processes, for example, it induces the inhibition of DNA repair and with this causes mutations. It also activates oncogenic pathways and alters the function of mitochondria.

When arsenic binds to certain sulfhydryl groups such as proteins, glutathione and cysteine affects the enzymes involved in cellular respiration, gluconeogenesis, glucose uptake and glutathione metabolism.

Arsenic creates resistance to apoptosis which is the process of programmed cell death carried out during the early stages of development to eliminate unnecessary cells. It is also believed to be responsible for aberrations and chromosomal abnormalities.

Unfortunately, arsenic is found in massive quantities in our cities, to the point that in countries such as China, India, Mexico, Thailand, the United States and Argentina there have been reports of chronic exposure to drinking water and it is estimated that in Latin America 4,5 Millions of people permanently drink water with alarming levels of this metal.

With this toxic metal that abounds in our planet, we finish our list of the most common endocrine disruptors in our day to day and therefore we are prepared to deepen the effects they have on health and the main diseases they generate.

Part III Effects on human health

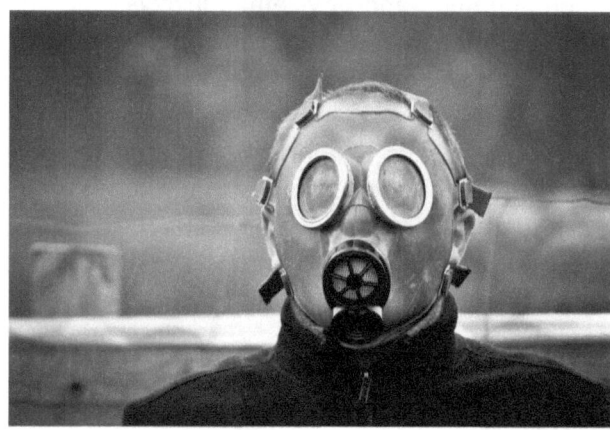

Chapter 22. Obesity

In medical terms, obesity is an excessive and widespread accumulation of fat in the body. It is a chronic pathology that in addition to affecting the appearance of the person increases the risk of contracting heart disease, diabetes and blood pressure, it also becomes a complicating factor of other health conditions such as arthritis.

The obesity rate today is alarming. It is estimated that approximately 22% of Spanish adults and 17% of children suffer from clinically detected obesity, while around 60% of adults worldwide suffer from overweight or obesity.

The distribution of the obese population is not uniform but we can detect a certain pattern. 50% is distributed in developed countries such as the United States, Mexico, Germany, United Kingdom, Brazil, Chile and Turkey, that is, developed countries are the most affected.

Why is obesity?

It is common to initially associate obesity and overweight with food and poor physical activity, but in reality it is only one of the many possible causes.

An unbalanced diet that exceeds the intake of calories in relation to physical activity, inevitably generates in the body the transformation of energy into fat stores and therefore, you can see an increase in weight in the person, but when a Patient leads a healthy lifestyle should evaluate other factors.

Some drug treatments, stress, lack of sleep or trying to quit smoking significantly increases the risk of obesity, also some stages such as menopause and postpartum.

Certain diseases such as Prader-Willi syndrome, Cushing syndrome and hormonal problems are also responsible for weight gain in the person, as well as genetic influences that can represent 60% of the risk of obesity.

Obesogens

Several chemicals that we have discussed in this book cause changes in metabolism that lead to weight gain, are called obesogens and have the property of altering adipogenesis and lipid accumulation.

Cigarette smoke, tributyltin, flame retardants, phthalates, bisphenol, parabens and organochlorine compounds are substances declared obesogenic and experts say they can act in three different ways in the body:

1.- Modifying the dynamics of fat cells: These substances can increase the fat storage capacity of the cells or increase their number and therefore the body's capacity.

2.- Altering the amount of calories consumed: If the substance alters the energy balance decreases the amount of calories consumed and favors the accumulation of fat.

3.- Altering the feeling of hunger: Hunger and the feeling of being satisfied are regulated by hormones and once they are unbalanced by external agents they cause the person constant states of hunger that lead him to overeat.

How to avoid obesogens?

Tributyltin, phthalates, bisphenol and organochlorine compounds are present both in controllable environments by us and in places that escape from our hands, so exposure in a certain way is inevitable.

Our attention and efforts should focus on minimizing our daily exposure, which is the aspect we can handle and represents a constant exposure factor. The measures you must take are the following:

- **Avoid plastic:** Bisphenol and phthalates are incorporated into the manufacture of plastics, but they are not fixed to the other substances but are released with heat and use and pass into the food and liquids they contain, so a measure Protective is to use glass containers and avoid using the microwave oven at all costs.

- **Buy products with the minimum amount of packaging:** Meats, fruits and vegetables that are packed in plastic are also exposed to contamination with obesogens. You can ask that the plastic be replaced by paper.

- **Check the origin of the food:** Call the companies whose products you usually buy and ask them to give you information on the origin of the food, if they are aware of the risks of exposure and the preventive measures they use.

- **Minimizes the use of creams and cosmetic products:** Parabens are present in the vast majority of creams, fixatives and makeup, so reduce their use only to what is necessary. Another alternative is to buy paraben-free products.

The most important effect of obesity is that it accentuates and aggravates in the short and long term other diseases such as diabetes, hypertension, some types of cancer and heart disease. In addition to affecting the patient's self-esteem and lifestyle.

Chapter 23. Metabolic syndrome

Also known as plurimetabolic syndrome or syndrome X, it is a group of disorders that occur at the same time in the patient and increase the probability of developing heart disease, suffering a stroke or suffering from type 2 diabetes.

A person with metabolic syndrome may experience an increase in blood pressure, high blood glucose levels, excess body fat (especially around the waist) and abnormal cholesterol or triglyceride levels.

The average age at which the disease appears is between 45 and 60 years and in 52.5% of the cases the affected patients are men. Likewise, people with some pathologies are more likely to develop the metabolic syndrome.

Cardiovascular disease, for example, increases the overall risk by 32%, only in men it reaches up to 45.2% and 17% in women. It seems that having one of the symptoms involves potentially exposing yourself to the rest, as diabetes and obesity also greatly increase the likelihood of developing the metabolic syndrome.

Causes

Many health specialists attribute the metabolic syndrome to overweight, obesity and lack of physical activity, others instead believe that insulin resistance is responsible.

Insulin is a hormone that is generated in the pancreas and is involved in the entry of glucose into cells to produce energy. When a person has insulin resistance, glucose cannot easily enter the cell membrane, so the blood glucose level increases and with this the insulin level rises to try to control the excess.

In other words, an imbalance is generated in the metabolic pathways that the organism uses to obtain, store and distribute energy.

The metabolic syndrome and endocrine disruptors

In a study published in the journal Environmental Science & Technology, 400 people living in Granada were monitored for ten years to determine if exposure to contaminants such as organochlorine compounds, bisphenol A, phthalates and perfluorinated compounds causes alterations.

The results of extensive research showed that exposure to organochlorine pesticides, even in relatively low doses, for a long time, increases the risk of metabolic syndrome and to a lesser extent industrial substances such as bisphenol A, phthalates and perfluorinated compounds.

The foundation of the research is that these substances create disorders and alterations in the energy balance of the organism, which is mainly controlled by signals from the endocrine system.

The most revealing part of the research is that it is presumed that these disorders may have their origin during prenatal development, and can be greatly influenced during postnatal development and adulthood.

What can we do to prevent it?

In Spain, one in two fresh vegetables is impregnated with at least one pesticide and a wide variety of fruits or vegetables can have 3 to 7 different pesticides.

Tomatoes, for example, are the most contaminated foods because they contain 37 different pesticides of which sixteen have hormonal effects. One of the most frequent chemicals in food is chlorpyriform, which has been found in 20 different foods throughout Spain, from potatoes and carrots to honey.

Since in this case food seems to be the greatest source of endocrine disruptors and it is illogical to eliminate them from our lives, the most successful alternative is to opt for ecological options, where the use of pesticides is practically non-existent.

Today there are many companies worldwide dedicated to the production of natural foods, both fruits, vegetables and cereals, as well as special baby foods, which are very vulnerable to contamination through intake.

Spain serves as a reference to demonstrate food contamination, which has a global reach. Nowadays it is necessary that you verify the origin of the fruits and vegetables that you consume, because the traditional industry has no alternatives but chemical weapons against pests and insects.

Chapter 24. Type 1 diabetes

Type 1 diabetes (DMT1) is a chronic disease whose onset usually takes place in childhood and adolescence, is characterized by a permanent and progressive elevation of blood sugar levels, that is, blood sugar levels, accompanied by destruction Autoimmune beta (β) cells of the islets of pancreatic Langerhans, which are responsible for the production of insulin.

DMT1 is considered to be an autoimmune disease and the causes of its occurrence are inconclusive, but its incidence globally has quite evident variations. The disease is less frequent in the regions located in the tropics, but it is more pronounced in the temperate regions, with a greater number of patients in the northern hemisphere than in the south. Approximately 1.25 million American children and adults have type 1 diabetes.

What originates it?

It is not known exactly the reason why type 1 diabetes appears, it is usually attributed to genetics but the fact of inheriting the genes of diabetes is often not an essential requirement to develop the disease.

The risk of developing DMT1 increases with the genetic transmission of the HLA DR3 and DR4 antigens, but the siblings of a child with the disease have only a 5% chance of developing it.

Scientists believe that genetic predisposition combined with external agents such as early exposure to cow's milk, stress, viruses and especially toxins found in currently used pesticides has more influence.

Pesticides and type 1 diabetes

A group of scientists from Greece and the United Kingdom have determined that eating food contaminated with pesticides can increase the risk of diabetes by up to 61% and that it reaches 64% when it is only type 2 diabetes.

To demonstrate this, the blood and urine results of 5,066 patients and 61,648 control cases were analyzed, which made the study a great medical evidence of how chemicals can promote the development of various pathologies.

On the other hand, a study presented at the annual congress of the European Association for the Study of Diabetes (EASD) showed that the exposure of pregnant women to certain common pesticides increases the probability of suffering from gestational diabetes fourfold.

The fruits and vegetables that we consume daily are contaminated and although they are essential for our health, the current conditions do not guarantee our well-being through food, so we will explore the alternatives we have to feed ourselves properly.

Consume only organic

The only really effective solution to avoid pesticides in food is simply to buy food free of the substance. Washing fruits, vegetables and vegetables with water from the jet is not as effective as we would like it to be.
Pesticides are designed and prepared not to dissolve easily in water, otherwise irrigation water and rains would end the

efficiency of the substance and would be a waste of money for the industry, so washing food only ends up with bacteria and remains of earth.

Other alternatives that are suggested are to eliminate the peel of the fruits, but this option is not appropriate for two reasons. In the first place the shell stores important amounts of nutrients and not consuming it is a waste and secondly the most toxic substances completely permeate the plant tissue.

Researchers at the Connecticut Agricultural Experimentation Station in the United States concluded after analyzing 196 samples of lettuce, tomatoes and strawberries that drying food with a cloth is more efficient for removing substances, but other experts say the solution lies in testing With baking soda.

An experiment carried out at the University of Massachusetts involved spraying apples with very penetrating fungicides and insecticides and then washing the fruits only with water, with a solution of bleach and bicarbonate dissolved in water. By keeping the apples submerged for two minutes in dissolved bicarbonate, more insecticides were suppressed than when they remained in the lye or in the water and it was the most efficient method to remove all types of waste, even dirt.

These practices could be a complementary measure to treat the foods we consume at home, but the option to buy organic foods remains more efficient.

Chapter 25. Type 2 diabetes

Type 2 diabetes is a chronic disease that affects the mechanism through which the body metabolizes glucose, that is, sugar. In the organism of the affected patient two things can happen, the first one is a resistance to the effects of insulin and the second the insufficient production of this hormone.

Unlike type 1 diabetes, the body produces insulin but does not use it properly and this disease was previously associated with adulthood, however, in the last decade there are numerous cases of children with the pathology due to the increase in obesity and sedentary lifestyle .

The World Health Organization (WHO) estimates that today approximately 442 million adults have diabetes, that is, one in 11 people and by 2015 it was estimated that diabetes was the direct cause of 1.6 million deaths.

This disease, so common in our society, is also one of the most worrisome, because in many affected people it is a cause of blindness, strokes, amputations, kidney failure, myocardial infarctions, gum and tooth problems. One of the biggest complications of diabetes is that in most cases it is diagnosed when it has several years of evolution and irreversible effects have already appeared in the patient.

Potential risks for a mother

In the previous chapter we saw that exposure to pesticides increases by 61% the probability of developing one of the two existing types of diabetes and also, that these probabilities increase when it is only type 2 diabetes, so we dedicate several indications to care of food, but pesticides are not solely responsible for diabetes.

Ángel Nadal, from the Miguel Hernández de Elche University, explains that each endocrine disruptor that circulates in the blood plasma with the capacity to produce insulin resistance can be considered a risk factor for metabolic syndrome and type 2 diabetes. Thus, Pesticides and other disruptors previously mentioned in the book are a threat but among this extensive list scientists have set their attention to one of fairly common use, BPA or bisphenol-A.

The Bioengineering Research Institute of the Miguel Hernández University of Elche discovered through its studies that exposure to bisphenol during pregnancy caused a profound alteration in glucose tolerance and worsens insulin resistance in the mother.

The investigation was carried out in female mice and it was observed that the metabolic alterations experienced were minimized after birth but four months later they were activated again and once they reached six months there was a marked decrease in insulin sensitivity, overweight and glucose intolerance.

It seems that BPA lowers insulin receptor levels, inhibits the phosphorylation of AKT and alters certain proteins, which results in resistance to insulin activity.
This fact adds one more concern for mothers: to compromise their own health during pregnancy. Thus, one of the precautions to be taken at this stage of life is to avoid exposure to bisphenol A

How to avoid bisphenol?

Bisphenol is present in plastic wrappings, toys, soft drink containers, food storage containers, resins and cans, which are elements of our daily use.

A mother in gestation should avoid or minimize as much as possible contact with plastics and canned foods, remember that the main route of contamination is through intake.

Substituting plastic for glass and buying fresh food instead of packaged or canned food is a simple measure that can be taken by mothers and in general anyone, to prevent the entry of the substance into the body. With small changes we can limit our exposure to hazardous chemicals in the environment that we are able to control.

Chapter 26. Hypothyroidism

Hypothyroidism, also known as underactive thyroid is a metabolic disorder in which the thyroid gland does not produce enough of certain crucial hormones, for example those that are related to caloric burning rate, body temperature or rapid heartbeat. cardiac

The disease does not show acute symptoms in the early stages but eventually triggers obesity, infertility, joint pain and certain heart diseases. In pregnancy it can be particularly dangerous for the baby in formation.

Around 700 million people worldwide suffer from some type of thyroid disorder, which is equivalent to 10% of the population or what is the same to say that at least three out of ten people have a health problem associated with the thyroid.

What causes hypothyroidism?

This disorder can be the product of an autoimmune disease, radiation therapy and certain medications, but it can also be generated through treatments for hyperthyroidism, which is thyroid overactivity.

In some newborn children, the thyroid may have low activity or may be born without it, in this case it is considered that they inherited the disorder. During pregnancy some women may develop the disease, both before and after, because hormonal changes generate antibodies that attack their own thyroid gland in an autoimmune response.

A disorder of the pituitary gland can also generate hypothyroidism but this cause is less frequent, it consists in the low production of thyrotropin (TSH), a thyroid stimulating hormone.

Of course, endocrine disruptors play an important role in thyroid activity, so we will now know their mechanism of action and what are the chemical substances responsible.

The role of thyroid disruptors

The mechanism through which substances such as PCBs (polychlorinated biphenyls) affect the thyroid is very simple to understand, basically they act as antagonists blocking hormone receptors and with this their metabolic and therapeutic action, also affecting brain cells.

Polychlorobiphenyls have been banned for a long time, but the chemical agent continues in the atmosphere and pollutes the bodies of water and the species that live there, as happens in French Brittany, where fish with a significant percentage of adipose tissue store easily the substance.

Pesticides also play an important role, as evidenced by a study carried out in Colombia, in South America, where it was intended to demonstrate the relationship between hypothyroidism and levels of organochlorine pesticides in blood, for this they studied 819 people residing in a rural area, of which 58.7% were men and 41.3% women.

In their results they obtained that the prevalence of overt hypothyroidism was 1.2% and 6.7% subclinical hypothyroidism, with the first percentage prevailing in people over 60 years of age, but without appreciable distinction in terms of sex.

There is a lot of evidence that shows how much our body chemicals can affect, in the case of PCBs and certain organochlorine pesticides directly affect one of the most important hormonal regulators, so preventive measures must be urgent.

How to take precaution against PCB?

Polychlorobiphenyls are present in dielectric fluids, heat exchangers and capacitors, metal carvings and turbine lubricants. In order for contamination with the substance to occur, some of the aforementioned devices must be damaged and come into contact with the soil and rainwater, thus reaching food and drinking water.

The first preventive measure to consider is to protect the equipment and devices in case you work with them or are close to your home, in case of an accident the affected area should be treated and avoided.

From home we can reduce the consumption of fish and food of animal origin if we are aware that in our region the risk of contamination with PCB is high, since the substance is stored without remedy in animal tissues.

If you live in a rural area or frequent it, protect your skin from mud, sediments, rivers and streams that could be contaminated and absorbed through the skin. If they draw water from a well with an old pump, check the appliance and investigate if it contains oil with PCBs, if so, you should change it.

TVs and refrigerators manufactured before 1980, as well as fluorescent tube reactances contain polychlorinated biphenyl in the condensers and for disposal they require a special process in which the substance is subtracted. It cannot be done at home.

With sufficient precautions we can keep ourselves protected from this substance, we must only remain attentive to our contact with ancient artifacts and the places we frequent.

Chapter 27. Thyroid Cancer

Thyroid cancer is a type of cancer that has as its place of origin the thyroid gland. This gland is located in the front of the neck, just below Adam's apple, but it is usually neither visible nor palpable.

Cancer, regardless of its location, originates when cells grow out of control and thyroid cancer is no exception, it is caused by an exacerbated cell growth of any type of cells that make up the gland. Depending on the cell is the type of disease that develops and therefore the treatment that the patient requires.

A thyroid gland can develop various types of growths and tumors, some are benign, but others unfortunately not and can spread to nearby tissues and other parts of the body.

For this year 2019 the American Cancer Society estimates 52,070 new cases of thyroid cancer, which 14,260 will be male patients, 37,810 women and 2% will occur in children and adolescents. On the other hand, it assumes that 2,170 people will die from the disease.

The mortality rate of thyroid cancer is low compared to other types of cancer, but in recent years it has experienced a significant increase.

Causes of the disease

The development of cancer is attributed to many causes, for example, exposure to certain chemicals, unhealthy habits and genetic load, the latter being the reason most limited by scientists around the world.

Genes contain very precise instructions to control when cells grow, divide and die, but for various reasons genes can encode uncontrolled cell growth and division or make these cells live longer than they should in a normal process. These genes are known as "oncogenes."

Cancer of any kind can be caused by modifications in the DNA that activate these "oncogenes" or by the deactivation of the genes that are responsible for suppressing errors.

Disruptors and thyroid

It is known that endocrine disruptors seriously interfere with thyroid functioning and in various ways. One of its effects is to generate changes in thyroid hormone concentrations, but it can also modify the peripheral metabolism of these hormones and receptor signaling.

Despite this knowledge, there is still a lack of information and evidence on how endocrine disruptors can affect the thyroid in very low concentrations, such as those we are exposed to daily by food, water and air. Some scientists explain that the disruptors cause cancer because they alter the normal homeostasis of the endocrine system and this results in an imbalance in the amount of estrogen, progestogen, androgen, and thyroid hormones. Others believe that these chemicals act as tumor promoters.

Today, the endocrine disruptors that have the most influence on the development of thyroid cancer are studied, however, halogenated organic compounds present in some pesticides have been suspected for more than a decade.

Halogenated substances have been responsible for alterations in the thyroid function of birds, fish and turtles, as well as dysfunctions in their immune system. This marks an important start for future studies on pathology.

Chapter 28. Breast Cancer

Breast cancer is a type of cancer that forms in breast tissue cells. It can occur in both women and men, although in the latter the breasts are not developed and do not fulfill any function in reproduction.

Thanks to the numerous investigations that have been carried out and the awareness campaigns worldwide, the disease survival rate is higher and today there are mechanisms for early detection and specialized treatments.

Doctors and scientists estimate that between 5% and 10% of breast cancer cases are related to inherited genetic mutations and for this year alone in the United States it is estimated that 271,270 people will be diagnosed, of which 268,600 cases will be women and 2,670 men

The female survival rate for metastatic breast cancer is 27% projected at 5 years, that is, 27 out of 100 people will survive more than this time, in men the rate is slightly lower, reaches 25%.

What causes breast cancer?

The disease develops when a group of mammary cells grow, divide abnormally and accumulate forming a lump or mass. Breast cancer usually begins in the cells of the ducts that produce breast milk or in the glandular tissue called the lobe.
Several studies show that there is a relationship between pathology and hormones, lifestyle and environment, however, a cause is not known exactly or why some women who apparently do not have any risk factor become patient Oncological

The great risk of breast cancer is that cells can spread throughout the breast tissue to the lymph nodes that are very close and from there to other parts of the body.

Disruptors and the disease

Although the exact causes of the development of the pathology are not known, there is evidence that some endocrine disruptors such as dichloro diphenyl trichloroethane (DDT) and dioxins have some responsibility.

The Journal of the National Cancer Institute published a study in which this relationship was discovered by studying exposed girls before the age of 14, who had a higher risk of developing cancer between 50 and 54 years of age, that is, in the premenopausal period.

In experimental animals it has been observed that particularly bisphenol A and dioxins are the breast cancer promoting substances. We already know the measures to avoid and minimize bisphenol, now it is the turn of dioxins.

How are dioxins controlled?

Controlling dioxins is very difficult for us because they come from industrial incineration and waste oils with PCBs, two processes regulated by private companies or government entities.

There are both national and international policies for the management of the substance and it is the duty of each country to carry out compliance, the only thing we can do on our own is to take care of the food that is a form of income.

Dioxins enter the environment and pass into the food chain, where we are consumers, therefore, we must take care of the intake of fatty foods, dairy and vegetables if we are aware that dioxins are a threat in our locality.

Chapter 29. Polycystic Ovarian Syndrome

Polycystic ovary syndrome, the acronym SOP, is a disorder present in women who have very high levels of a hormone called androgen. Both men and women naturally have androgen, but the tendency in the male gender is to maintain a high level, when this occurs in a female, some complications appear.

Menstrual irregularities, increased facial hair, the appearance of acne and infertility are some symptoms of PCOS, as well as the growth of ovarian cysts, but they are only noticeable by medical procedures.

One in ten women of childbearing age suffer from polycystic ovary syndrome, that is, 10% of the female population between the ages of 15 and 44. 10% of infertile patients have follicular cysts in their ovaries.

Why does PCOS develop?

Usually, a patient with PCOS has a direct relative who also suffers from it, so the genetic predisposition for the disorder is undeniable, but there is not enough evidence to support that it is the only cause.

Polycystic ovary syndrome is diagnosed in women whose age ranges between 20 or 30 years, but it can appear in girls and adolescents, in any case it is the product of a hormonal imbalance.

When androgen levels rise to estrogen, and progesterone drops and these hormones are involved in the maturation and release of the ovules during ovulation. When PCOS is suffered, mature ovules are not released and instead remain in the ovaries covered by fluid, this is why cysts and bulges are generated in the ovaries.

Early diagnosis and treatment compliance normalize the symptoms of the disorder and prevent complications such as type 2 diabetes and heart disease, which are closely related.

How do disruptors influence PCOS?

According to various studies, endocrine disruptors and particularly bisphenol A are present in high concentrations in adolescents and adult women with PCOS, compared to healthy women. A higher incidence of hyperandrogenemia was also discovered, which clearly demonstrates the relationship of the effects on the endocrine system by the substance.

Thus, the scientists conclude that constant exposure to endocrine disruptors such as bisphenol will permanently alter neuroendocrine, reproductive and metabolic regulation, therefore favoring the development of PCOS in women with a genetic predisposition or that it may well accelerate and exacerbate symptoms in those They already suffer.

Bisphenol A is one of the biggest responsible for endocrine problems today due to its presence in plastic and the constant use of us with that material. One of the biggest concerns is that more recent animal studies show that reproductive function can be drastically altered by exposure in the perinatal period.

If polycystic ovarian syndrome is due to a disorder in the hormones involved in reproduction and endocrine disruptors affect precisely the hormonal center of our body, it is not surprising that 30% of clinically obese people and 10% of those Patients with diabetes have the disorder at some stage of their life.

Here we reflect once again the importance of reducing contact with plastic in our day to day. It is a measure that we have already mentioned in other chapters, however, given the consequences derived from bisphenol and other disruptors it is more than convenient to remember it.

Chapter 30. Early ovarian failure

Early ovarian failure, also known as premature ovarian failure (FOP) is a loss of normal ovarian function before reaching 40 years of age. It is characterized by deficiency in the production of estrogen, amenorrhea and female infertility.

Early ovarian failure is not the same as premature menopause, although they are often confused, in the first women have irregular or occasional menstrual periods for years and there is the possibility of pregnancy if proper treatment is carried out, premature menopause leads at the end of reproductive activity and therefore total disappearance of menstruation.

Statistically, one in every 100 women under 40 will suffer a premature ovarian failure and only one in ten thousand women in their twenties. Usually, helping the patient recover estrogen levels prevents complications such as osteoporosis, which occurs when the body maintains low estrogen levels.

What causes this disorder?

The cause of early ovarian failure is unknown in 90% of diagnosed cases. Medical advances establish that FOP develops when two types of problem appear in the ovarian follicles, which is the site where the ovules develop.

It can happen that the follicles stop working sooner than normal or they don't work well and prevent the development of the ovum. Certain genetic diseases, some metabolic disorders and treatments such as chemotherapy may be responsible for these two conditions in the ovary.

In recent years, the effect of some toxic substances, such as cigarette smoke and pesticides, has been evaluated, as there seems to be a relationship between their effect on health and the appearance of FOP.

How do endocrine disruptors influence?

Certain metals such as cadmium and nickel, solvents and pesticides, can affect ovarian function by triggering a hormonal or autoimmune disorder, or induce cell proliferation and accelerated apoptosis.

Scientists believe that the effect of the disruptors occurs through estrogen receptors and aromatic hydrocarbon receptors, giving rise to three different mechanisms of action.

First, follicular atresia (decrease) can be generated during ovule growth thanks to an increase in oxidative stress and apoptosis. They could also alter the signaling pathways influencing folliculogenesis and finally there is the possibility of modifications in the DNA that alter the ovarian function.

Folliculogenesis begins in fetal development and it is thought that environmental exposure and the lifestyle of the parent can trigger these types of problems and some similar, however, evidence is still sought to confirm transgenerational inheritance of FOP when it comes from contamination environmental.

How to avoid heavy metals?

Metals such as nickel and cadmium, can be found in food, but also in the utensils we use, stainless steel pots, for example, release small particles of the substance as it is used and exposed to heat, therefore Our prevention measure must revolve around limiting its use and obtaining other alternatives to prepare food.

Avoiding cigarettes and passive smoking, is another effective way to avoid exposing ourselves to cadmium and nickel, as tobacco plants absorb the substance from the earth, passes to the cigarette and are released into the atmosphere in the combustion process.

Reducing and completely eliminating contact with heavy metals during pregnancy can prevent serious diseases in the baby, therefore, we must pay attention to fruits, vegetables and fish, which are the most common sources of metals in the diet.

Chapter 31. Ovarian Cancer

Ovarian or ovarian cancer is a type of cancer that originates in the ovaries. A woman's reproductive system has two ovaries, one on each side of the fallopian tubes and is responsible for producing eggs and hormones such as estrogen and progesterone.

When the cells in this region of the body begin to grow out of control, the disease originates, which is not very easy to detect at an early stage, in fact, only in 20% of cases a detection is made in the early stages and patients more frequent are elderly women, that is, women over sixty.

This disease is the second most common in gynecology and by 2019 the American Cancer Society estimates that in the United States there will be about 22,530 new diagnoses and approximately 13,980 deaths.

The risk of any woman suffering from the disease is 78%, this means that every 78 females one will be affected and their probability of dying is one in one hundred and eight, regardless of benign ovarian tumors that do not represent a risk.

Thanks to medical and scientific advances the chances of surviving ovarian cancer the survival rate is 44% over a period of five years, regardless of age, stage or histological type. Survival is much higher in germ cell tumors and carcinomas, is close to 90% and has more diagnosis in adolescents and young people.

What disruptors are responsible?

Many endocrine disruptors on the list are considered potentially dangerous because they are tumor promoters or cause alterations in cellular behavior, but some parts of the body appear more vulnerable than others to exposure to the substance.

Pesticides, for example, like plasticizers such as bisphenol A, phthalates, dioxins, polychlorinated biphenyls and polycyclic aromatic hydrocarbons are associated with ovarian cancer because they can alter the synthesis and metabolism of ovarian steroid sex hormones and this generates important imbalances.

What is your mecanism of action?

Endocrine disruptors act as estrogenic or as androgenic, but regardless of their behavior, both can cause endocrine alterations in the ovaries by binding to estrogen (RE) or androgen (RA) receptors and interfering with the action of endogenous steroid hormones.

A disruptor does not act in a single way, it actually has several alternatives for example, altering the expression or enzymatic activity necessary for the synthesis or degradation of sex steroids or modifying the expression of hormone receptors and their ability to bind to their ligands

In an "in vitro" study with ovarian cancer cells it was discovered that xenoestrogen 1 bisphenol A, which has a chemical structure similar to 17β-estradiol (E2) and is naturally present in the female body, has an estrogenic effect on the Induction of apoptosis, cell cycle and cancer genes has also been shown that a high expression of ER-α receptors compared to normal tissue increases the chances of disease.

92

Female health, due to its creative capacity for life and its endocrine dependence, seems to be more vulnerable to the effect of endocrine disruptors, since we have already seen four different pathologies specific to this genus and there are still some more. This is one of the main reasons that led us to write this book: the urgency of taking measures for health and well-being.

Chapter 32. Female Infertility

Infertility or female infertility is the difficulty in achieving or maintaining a pregnancy. It is a condition that has experienced an increase in recent years and may be due to multiple factors.

Menstrual disorders such as anovulation, endometriosis, abnormalities of the fallopian tubes or uterus, cervical mucus problems, serious diseases, age, weight and stress are the main causes of this condition in a woman, but there are also patients who present an infertility inexplicable and others whose problem is caused by exposure to endocrine disruptors.

In medical terms, a couple is considered sterile when they try unsuccessfully to conceive a baby for a period of one year or more. Worldwide it is estimated that between 10-18% of couples have some type of problem to reach a successful delivery, but it is not always due to female problems.

About a third of the time infertility in a couple is due to female aspects, a third to male factors and another third to a combination of common factors between both or indeterminate causes, so in recent years assisted reproduction treatments have increased.

In Spain alone, approximately 50,000 in vitro fertilization treatments and almost 30,000 artificial inseminations are done annually. It is strong evidence that something is affecting the reproductive health of our society, as well as the fact that 3% of Spanish babies are born by assisted reproduction techniques according to the medical director of the IVI group, Antonio Requena.

Endocrine disruptors and female infertility

The effect of a disruptor on female fertility is very varied because not all substances act in the same way and are not the direct cause, but infertility is a consequence of its action on the reproductive system and the endocrine system, such as We show in the following paragraphs.

Bisphenol A: Present in cans, plastics and bottles, this disruptor decreases the quality of the ovarian reserve, negatively influences during embryonic implantation and the development of the fetus.

Triclosan: This antiseptic product significantly decreases the quality of the oocyte, which is the immature form of an ovule and with this decreases the possibility of a conception.

PFC or perfluorinated: They are usually used as waterproof and non-stick and significantly reduce the pregnancy rate and increase the risk of a miscarriage.

Pesticides: Pesticides increase the number of abortions and ectopic pregnancies, in which embryo implantation takes place outside the uterus and therefore is not feasible.

Polychlorinated biphenyls: This substance that was formerly used in machinery and certain electronic components generates endometriosis and a decrease in antimullerian hormone (HAM) levels that determines the quantity and quality of ovarian follicles in a woman.

Heavy metals also influence female fertility by increasing the risk of abortion, that is, they prevent the successful completion of a pregnancy. Thus, the behavior of the disruptors in our body is unpredictable because it can cause a pathology or limit our reproductive capacity, but not only that, the health of the baby is also at risk.

Recall that many of these disruptors are responsible for genetic mutations and some disorders that we will discuss later in this book.

Chapter 33. Endometriosis

Endometriosis is a condition in which endometrial tissue grows outside the uterus unpredictably, being able to lodge on the peritoneum, ovaries, intestines, fallopian tubes, bladder, skin or lungs, but these last two sites are less frequent.

Although the endometrial tissue is lodged in a different place to the uterus, it reacts together with the hormones of the menstrual cycle and bleeds, but the flow in other parts of the body does not have an escape route and generates inflammation, pain and internal scars in the affected patient.

When the endometrial tissue grows in the ovaries the blood can become embedded and form fibrous cysts and when located between organs it can cause adhesion and therefore pain.

The exact causes that cause endometriosis are unknown but one of the possible reasons is that when a woman has the period, a retrograde flow develops by which the cells travel through the fallopian tubes and return to the pelvis. Some specialists say that the disease develops as a result of a failure in the immune system, for others instead it is genetics and it is thought that it can be transmitted from one generation to another.

If we review the world statistics we will realize that the pathology is a factor that influences fertility, because between 24% and 50% women who have endometriosis have difficulty conceiving a child and that it is a recurring disease in the United States , where it is estimated that more than 5 million women are affected.

Why is endometriosis generated?

When endometriosis appears there is a failure in female steroid hormones, that is, estrogen and progesterone that are responsible for regulating endometrial growth by stimulation or cell proliferation.

To carry out its function, estrogen must be linked to one of the estrogen receptors (ER), which can be ER-α or ER-β. Scientific studies in which the ectopic endometrial tissue (outside the uterus) was studied demonstrated the expression of estrogen receptors, mainly ER-α, so it is assumed that it is strongly related. The presence of aromatase, an enzyme that is responsible for producing estrogens, has also been found in endometrial tissue.

What is the role of disruptors?

The role of endocrine disruptors in the development of endometriosis is inconclusive, but there is evidence of its effect. In many studies the compounds were studied individually but no effect was found, however a synergistic effect was suspected, that is, by the sum of other factors, which was later demonstrated.

A medical study measured the level of substances considered disruptors in 84 women undergoing laparoscopy for endometriosis and 3.77 times higher levels were found compared to women without the pathology. Simply put, women with a high level of substances in the body were more likely to develop the disease.

The endocrine disruptors that are considered potentially responsible for the development of endometriosis have already been mentioned in this section of the book and we have explained how to avoid them, such as PCBs, perfluorinated compounds, pesticides, alkylphenols, parabens, bisphenol A and phthalates.

According to studies, none seems to be directly responsible, but all are at the moment they are in high proportions within the body, which is a bit more dangerous if you consider how difficult it is to control some substances mentioned

Chapter 34. Uterine Fibroids

Uterine fibroids, also known as myomas or leiomyomas, are benign tumors in the uterus that appear during the fertile age of women. Only 0.5% of myomas become malignant tumors or sarcomas, which is cancer that originates in muscle tissues, fat and bones.

A fibroid varies greatly in size, they can be very small and barely noticeable with sight or be very bulky and distort and enlarge the uterus. Similarly, only one or several may appear, grow over time or decrease in size. The formation of a uterine fibroid does not follow a pattern; it can merit years or develop rapidly in a short time.

Myomas are not very dangerous for female health, but they generate pain, infertility and heavy bleeding that can be controlled with proper treatment. In Europe, the annual amount of money invested in the treatment of this condition is alarming.

It is estimated that by 2016 the European continent spent 1.4 billion euros in medical treatment and loss of fertility caused by endometriosis and uterine fibroids, and according to the University of New York University School of Medicine the two diseases were caused by endocrine disruptors.

What happens in the rest of the world?

Europe has approximately 24 million affected and many of them do not consult a doctor until after five years according to the gynecologist and researcher of the Karolinska Institute, Helena Kopp. But this high rate is not exclusive to the region, worldwide 40% of women between 35 and 55 years have uterine fibroids.

This means that at the age of 45 years about 70% of women have developed at least one myoma but ignore it because in 30% of cases women do not present any symptoms immediately, so the time since The appearance of myoma until consultation with a doctor is not about carelessness on the part of the patient.

What causes fibroids?

The exact cause of the appearance of myomas is not known, but it is suspected that elevated levels of estrogen and possibly progesterone stimulate its growth.

During pregnancy, when estrogen and progesterone levels increase, myomas increase in size, but tend to become small after menopause, when their levels decrease due to the changes of that period, however, when the end of Reproductive age Women are at greater risk of developing a fibroid due to the production peaks that hormones experience.

Women who are obese and those of African-American descent are more likely to suffer from uterine fibroids, but at the medical level the reason has not been discovered.

Why are fibroids attributed to disruptors?

It is very likely that the appearance and growth of fibroids is controlled by hormones (estrogen and progesterone) and it is well known that endocrine disruptors have the power to prevent and modify the natural action of hormones and that their mechanism of action Once they enter the body it is unpredictable.

It is considered that the responsible disruptors could be phthalates, heavy metals, perfluorinated compounds and PCBs, but it is mainly attributed to the former.

In a European study in which the urine of 145,000 European women diagnosed with endometriosis and uterine fibroids was analyzed, a high level of phthalates was found in their samples, which leads doctors and scientists to reach this conclusion, however, also there is evidence that the other substances mentioned have an important influence.

Chapter 35. Recurring Abortions

Recurrent abortion is a consecutive and unplanned or induced pregnancy loss. A couple is considered to suffer from recurrent abortions when they experience three or more successive abortions before they reach twenty weeks of gestation.

Recurrent abortions are a multifactorial reproductive problem and it is difficult to determine because it affects a very heterogeneous population, that is, very varied.

Statistically, about 1 and 3% of couples of reproductive age lose an unexpected pregnancy, 15% of clinically recognized pregnancies end in abortions and 25% of women in general will experience an abortion at least once in his life.

The influence of endocrine disruptors on recurrent abortions is quite broad and complex because no single cause can be attributed, but to many factors that could affect both parents and the embryo.

Abortions caused by endocrine disruptors

In previous chapters we have explained some pathologies that develop in the female reproductive system thanks to the presence of a disruptive chemical agent, these diseases could become responsible for recurrent abortions in a woman, let's see below why:

Uterine fibroids: These benign tumors are believed to be caused by a lack of control of estrogen and progesterone levels. Here we find two possibilities for the loss of a pregnancy.

The hormonal balance is essential for a pregnancy to take place within the body, if a conception is achieved but the conditions are not suitable the embryo will not have a safe place to stay or protection and eventually the pregnancy will be lost. On the other hand, large myomas can distort the uterus and make the space for the embryo very small.

Chronic endometritis: Endometriosis also has hormonal causes, but instead of benign tumors, it usually causes intrauterine lesions and other parts of the pelvis, which present with bleeding and inflammation. Endometriosis is associated with aetiology of recurrent abortion between 5 to 27%.

Sperm involvement: In some cases the reason for recurrent abortions may not be in the mother but in the parent. The quality of the sperm that fertilizes the egg is essential to maintain a successful pregnancy.

The study of the male component in cases of recurrent losses showed that in these men the DNA damage was 16% higher compared to fertile men whose partner had no problems to conclude a pregnancy.

DNA fragmentation present in sperm is associated with numerous indicators of reproductive health, for example, embryonic quality, implantation, spontaneous abortion and congenital malformations.

Obesity, insulin resistance and polycystic ovary: Several authors affirm that these pathologies are related to an increased risk of spontaneous abortion due to the imbalance and modifications suffered by the organism, for example, women with insulin-dependent diabetes whose disease control

It is deficient have a 2 to 3 times higher abortion rate than non-diabetic women.

Thus, recurrent abortion is more complex than one might think. Unfortunately, diseases caused by endocrine disruptors are related in some way or another to the reproductive health of the parents or the normal development of an embryo.

With such high rates of polycystic ovary, obesity and diabetes, it is imperative to check our health before planning a family, because we now know that these medical conditions make the task of bringing a baby to the world more difficult.

Chapter 36. Intrauterine growth retardation

Delayed fetal growth or restricted intrauterine growth is a condition that causes the baby in formation to be smaller than expected for gestational age. When it occurs, the fetus does not grow inside the uterus at the rate it should and usually have a lower weight at birth.

At the level of obstetrics and pediatrics, these patients weigh less than the 10th percentile, that is, the baby weighs less than 9 out of 10 babies of the same age and this is a cause of concern for both parents and providers of Health carry the pregnancy.

Restriction of fetal growth can affect the overall size of the baby, but also the growth of organs, tissues and cells and this can cause problems before and after birth.

10% of cases of intrauterine growth retardation are related to specific gene abnormalities and congenital metabolism errors that cause pregnancy termination, for example, trisomy 15. Some syndromes such as Turner, Edwards and Beckwith-Wiedman are also responsible of slow fetal growth.

What complications does retarded growth bring?

A baby with restricted intrauterine growth may have breathing difficulties and infections. You may also need to be born earlier and stay in the hospital while your body reaches some stability and maturity.

Some pregnant women under this condition die before or after birth and a good percentage is exposed to acquiring heart and blood vessel problems.

For many health experts, the most common cause of fetal growth problems is the malfunction of the placenta, but it may also be due to exposure to X-rays, infections such as rubella, high blood pressure during pregnancy and smoking . The latter coincides with endocrine disruptors.

Endocrine disruptors and embryonic growth

Cadmium, which is one of the heavy metals that acts as disruptors of the endocrine system, is incorporated into the biomass of plants such as cocoa and tobacco and reach a person's body when they smoke.

Recall that when smoking is generated cadmium oxide that is absorbed by the body quickly and it is estimated that 50% of all the metal that is inhaled in this way enters the bloodstream, but can be avoided simply by quitting smoking and would bring large Benefits to the fetus

Pregnant women exposed to cadmium are more likely to experience spontaneous abortions and fetuses contaminated under birth weight, this is because the metal decreases the synthesis of leptin, a hormone that regulates organogenesis and fetal development.

On the other hand, it seems that the combination of multiple disruptors in the mother's organism dramatically increases the probability that fetal growth is retarded, as demonstrated by a study carried out by the Institute of Global Health of Barcelona.

The research results show that women with jobs classified as exposed to one or more groups of endocrine disruptors had a 25% higher risk of having a low weight baby and that the risk is proportional to the number of exposure substances, that is , it multiplies.

It is surprising to discover the various forms in the substances that we have seen in this book can affect our life, even before the moment of birth when our body is still in formation and we are not aware of what is happening.

Chapter 37. Preterm Birth

Premature or premature delivery occurs three weeks before the clinically scheduled date. A woman is considered to have a birth and a premature baby when the birth occurs before the 37th week of gestation.

The human pregnancy lasts 40 weeks from the first day of the last menstruation, which is equivalent to 9 months and is enough time for all the organs, systems and devices of the baby to complete their training and reach the maturity necessary to become independent of the umbilical cord , but when the delivery occurs early the baby has health problems.

According to statistics from the World Health Organization (WHO), 15 million premature children are born every year around the world, and unfortunately one million of them fail to survive because their body conditions do not allow it.

Preterm birth is a major cause of diseases (morbidity) and perinatal mortality, for example, the United States has an incidence of premature births of 12%, but if we exclude congenital malformations 75% of perinatal deaths and 50% Neurological problems are due to prematurity of the baby.

The premature baby can have a small size with a disproportionately large head, few fat reserves and therefore be thinner, breathing problems and few sucking reflexes, it can also be born covered with lanugo or fine hair.

What causes premature delivery?

The early birth of a baby may be due to an infection of the mother, kidney disease, obesity, heart or thyroid problems, diabetes or severe anemia, among many other diseases and disorders.

Other conditions such as being under 17 years of age or over 35, having previously suffered a premature birth, excessive physical activity, an abnormally shaped uterus, stress and depression are also responsible for early deliveries, but of course endocrine disruptors have An important paper.

Phthalates, bisphenol, biphenyls and premature deliveries

Thanks to various studies, scientists believe that exposure to phthalates, bisphenol, biphenyls, organochlorine pesticides and perfluorinated compounds increases the risk of premature delivery, but their action as a whole is considered more dangerous than that of each substance separately.

In a study by the University of Michigan, the urine of almost 500 pregnant women with premature births was analyzed for traces of phthalates and the results of the laboratory analysis were compared with the urine of women whose pregnancy culminated in the expected time, the amount of the substance was higher in the first group.

Another research conducted at the University of California, which appeared in the journal Environmental Health Perspectives, analyzed a total of 268 women participating in a national health survey and up to 163 different chemicals were detected in 99% of the participants.

Some of the substances that the scientists found were bisphenol-A, polychlorinated biphenyls, organochlorine pesticides, perfluorinated compounds, phenols, phthalates and polycyclic aromatic hydrocarbons, but more attention was given to Bisphenol A.

The conclusion of the study was that not all substances found in mothers are presented in amounts dangerous enough to affect pregnancy, but some of them in high amounts affect pregnancy significantly.

In addition, specialists point out that exposure to multiple substances may be more harmful to health than the impact that a single chemical could cause within the body.

These substances are linked to food and plastic and in previous chapters we have mentioned the necessary measures to avoid them. With the evidence that until the date of a delivery it can be affected by endocrine disruptors, it is an important fact to make forecasts before planning a family.

Chapter 38. Low birth weight

"Low birth weight" is the phrase used at the medical level when a baby is born weighing less than 5 pounds and 8 ounces. The World Health Organization (WHO) defines that a low birth weight is below 2,500 g.

Premature birth and restricted fetal growth, two conditions we saw earlier, are primarily responsible for a birth below normal weight. Some babies are healthy despite being thin and have no problems during their development, however, others have serious health problems.

A newborn baby with low body weight may have problems with feeding, normal weight gain that you should experience month to month and may have difficulty fighting infections.

If we review world statistics, we observe that between 15% and 20% of babies are below their normal weight, which is equivalent to 20 million infants per year. In the United States about 8% of births are underweight.

WHO aims to reduce the number of children with this problem by 30% by 2025. To achieve this, the rate must be reduced annually by 3% between 2012 and 2025, so the number of affected newborns would go from 20 million to 14 million

Why is a child born underweight?

Certain infections and especially genetic problems affect the organism of the developing baby so that your body does not develop as it should and can make it smaller and thinner than it should at the time of birth. It also affects pregnancy, a fetus with congenital problems is more likely to be born before a fetus that does not have them.

The mother's habits also influence the weight a baby can gain during pregnancy. Smoking, drinking alcohol and using illegal drugs are practices that affect fetal development and retard its growth, increasing the chances of premature birth and therefore a poor birth weight.

Of course there are environmental factors associated with the low in infants, especially exposure to disruptors present in flame retardants, perfluoroalkylated chemicals and lead, which are involved in fetal development to a point that seriously limit their growth.

Lead and low birth weight

High levels of lead in a pregnant woman can cause miscarriages and lifeless births, but in other cases it can lead to premature birth and low birth weight. Other effects that could be found in a child born under these conditions are learning and behavior problems.

Recall that lead is associated with cognitive problems in young children, intoxication due to the difficulty of their body to bear harmless doses for adults and malformations, so when it comes to babies and young children extra protection measures should be taken against this substance.

What to do to avoid exposure to lead?

A mother who suspects that lead exposure can affect her pregnancy can take the following steps when planning to create her family:

- Have a blood test to detect blood metal levels and check that it is suitable or not for a healthy pregnancy.

- Avoid painting the baby's room with lead-based paints and before, during and after pregnancy, do not expose yourself to this product.

- Request information from the distributors of drinking water about the water treatment that comes to your home.

- Make several meals a day. Lead from the environment is more easily absorbed through the bloodstream and remains more in the body when the stomach is empty.

- Eat a diet low in calcium, iron, zinc, vitamin C, vitamin D and vitamin E that are associated with the growth of the amount of lead that is absorbed into your bloodstream.

Chapter 39. Early loom

The development of breast tissue in a girl with an age less than 8 years is called early telarchy or early loom. The appearance of the breast button is usually the first visible sign of puberty in girls and occurs due to an increase in estrogen, but under normal conditions it must occur between 11 and 16 years.

The early loom is not synonymous with precocious puberty although in healthy girls the loom is the beginning of puberty. There are girls whose breast button appears several years before menarche or first menstruation and pubarche, which is the appearance of pubic hair.

The annual incidence of this disorder in girls is 1 in 5000, in other words, every year one in 5000 girls is diagnosed with early loom, but in 60% of cases the patient is less than 2 years old and mostly condition occurs from the moment of birth.

In 85% of girls who have early telarchy it is a benign and self-limited disorder called "isolated benign telarchy" and will not be a serious problem for the little one since it can lead to normal development for her age and will not have an early puberty, but it must remain under the supervision of a pediatrician.

Only 15% of girls have precocious puberty and other sexual characters appear prematurely, such as axillary and pubic hair or vaginal bleeding.

Chemical substances associated with early loom

There are three substances with an endocrine disruptor effect that are associated with the early appearance of the breast button in girls, these are: phthalates, phytoestrogens and lavender. Phthalates, which have an antiandrogenic effect, are found in plastic toys, children's hygiene products, cosmetics and in patients with early loom a higher concentration of metabolites of this substance has been observed compared to girls without any disorder.

Similarly, products such as pesticides, herbicides and derivatives of the chemical industry also induce the early development of the breasts through a direct activity towards the estrogen receptor, or through an increase in the activity of the aromatase enzyme, which generates an increase in glandular volume.

We know perfectly well how to avoid phthalates and these measures are applicable to children, however the other two substances have not been mentioned in the book. Phytoestrogens are present in soybeans and all products obtained from it and lavender is a common plant that has an effect on the endocrine system.

Phytoestrogens are compounds of estrogenic activity that are found naturally in plants and foods, particularly in soybeans. A girl whose diet rich in this type of food is exposed to suffering from early loom due to the effects of the substance on her body.

Lavender for its part is integrated into various cosmetic products such as body creams and shampoos, but this substance has estrogenic properties and antiandrogenic activities, which means that it competes or hinders hormones that control male characteristics, which could affect puberty and growth

How to avoid the early loom?

Early loom can be prevented by restricting a girl's exposure to phthalates, phytoestrogens and lavender. You can replace most of your plastic toys with others made of a different material such as wood, provided that resins or plasticizers are not used to protect them.

The material with which your bottle, glass and cutlery is made is also important, there are several companies that are dedicated to the manufacture of products for babies free of harmful chemicals.

The consumption of soy and its products should be regulated by a pediatrician and nutritionist so that if the family consumes the food regularly, the child is not affected.

Finally there is lavender, a substance that can be easily avoided if you buy products free of it. These measures are easy to carry out but very effective to take care of the health and proper development of a girl.

Chapter 40. Precocious female puberty

At the clinical level it is considered that a girl goes through an early puberty when the first physical changes of adulthood appear before her age before 8 years, this includes aspects related to sexual development.

In girls the first pubertal pattern is breast development, then the appearance of pubic hair and axillary hair takes place and finally the first menstruation arrives, which occurs between two and four years after the loom and usually occurs between 12 and 16 years.

Precocious puberty seems to have a different incidence according to the genes of the affected girl, for example, in African descendants it appears in 20-30%, while in girls with Caucasian genes it occurs in 8-10% of the population.

There are two types of precocious puberty, one dependent on the gonadotropin-releasing hormone and another independent, they are known as central and peripheral precocious puberty respectively.

Gonadotropin-dependent precocious puberty (GnRH) occurs in both sexes and is 5 to 10 times more frequent in girls. In this disorder, it activates the hypothalamic-pituitary axis that determines the increase in size and maturation of the gonads, development of secondary sexual characteristics and oogenesis or spermatogenesis.

In the independent early puberty of GnRH, secondary sexual characteristics appear due to the high circulating concentrations of estrogens or androgens, but there is no activation of the hypothalamus-pituitary axis and therefore there is no maturation of the gonads.

What induces precocious puberty in girls?

There are many factors that can induce precocious puberty in girls, for example obesity and exposure to endocrine disruptors.

A recent study examined more than 1,100 girls at age 9 and then at age 26 and it was found that each increase in a standard deviation of the Body Mass Index (BMI) at the age of 9 was correlated with twice the possibilities of having menarche before 12. This is mainly due to a hormone called leptin that is produced by fatty tissue, inhibits appetite and promotes the release of kisspeptin, another hormone whose function is to stimulate the neurons responsible for activating the releasing hormone of gonadotrophins.

So the more fatty tissue a girl has, the higher the level of leptin and kisspeptin will have her body and therefore an earlier onset of puberty.

The effect of endocrine disruptors is now very specific thanks to the efforts of the National Institute of Environmental Health Sciences and the US Environmental Protection Agency. UU, which has clear evidence of which commonly used products and chemicals induce precocious puberty.

The scientists showed that antibacterial gels, personal care products and cleaning substances contain triclosan, phthalates, parabens and phenols, four substances that cause the early appearance of breasts, pubic hair and other characteristics of sexual development.

His study consisted of evaluating 179 girls and 159 boys. During the experiment they measured the concentrations of the four substances in the urine collected from the mothers during pregnancy and later that of the children when they reached 9 years of age. Puberty time was evaluated every 9 months between the ages of 9 and 13 years.

When analyzing the results, the scientists in charge of the investigation discovered that:

- The high level of triclosan in maternal urine during pregnancy could have a greater influence on the early onset of menstrual periods.

- The high level of phthalates in the mother's urine during pregnancy could accelerate the development of pubic hair.

- Girls with high levels of methylparaben or propylparaben in the urine had an early onset of menstruation, breast button and pubic hair compared to the other girls of their age.

- Girls with high levels of 2,5-dichlorophenol in the urine had a delayed development of pubic hair.

It has been shown that girls who experience precocious puberty have a higher risk of breast and ovarian cancer, in addition to their behavior and self-esteem being more affected than that of their peers.

These problems can be avoided with simple measures, such as avoiding exposure to plastic in both the mother and the child and reducing cosmetic and cleaning products to the essential, always preferring options free of hazardous chemicals.

Chapter 41. Small penis

Microfalosomy, Shadi's disease or micropene, is a penis with a very short length compared to an average male member. A small penis in a flaccid state is two centimeters and erect does not reach more than seven. There are some cases in which the male genital is barely visible, resembling more the female clitoris.

For socially imposed ideas many men consider that they have a small penis, but to determine a small penis at the medical level, the base is also considered, not just the free part.

In other words, a small penis with a maximum erection does not exceed eight centimeters from the pubic bone to the tip of the glans, with the foreskin retracted. In this way, only a small percentage of the world's male population is affected by this condition, 1 in 10,000 men.

Why is a child born with microfalosomy?

A small penis is the result of insufficient androgenic stimulation, which leads to delayed growth of the external genitalia in men. This condition can be caused by primary hypogonadism or hypothalamic or pituitary dysfunction.

Hypogonadism is a disorder in which the sexual characteristics of man are not well developed by late biological maturation, such as constitutional growth retardation, or by a testicular lesion that affects the production of testosterone and sperm, in this case it would be treated of hypergonadotropic hypogonadism.

Microfalosomy may also be due to alterations in meiosis, which is the process of cellular reproduction. In this case there is an inadequate differentiation of the Leydig cells, which are the producers of testosterone, the most important sex hormone in man and are located in the testicles.

Testosterone deficiency during pregnancy is one of the factors that are also responsible for the small size of a penis and other genital abnormalities. When the male fetus does not produce enough testosterone or the mother does not produce enough human chorionic gonadotrophin hormone, the male genitalia have difficulty developing.

Can disruptors cause a small penis?

Until recently there was no clear evidence that endocrine disruptors had any influence on the development of microfalosomy, in fact, this condition was attributed to congenital diseases and although there is a certain relationship it is not the only influencing factor.

A study published in the journal PLOS Computational Biology gathered and analyzed thousands of medical records from the United States in search of an answer for the high rate of autism and mental disabilities presented in some counties of the country.

The researchers found that both pathologies coincide geographically with the areas in which children have a high incidence of genital malformations. More specifically, boys with autism spectrum disorders were 5.53 times more likely to have genital malformations.

According to the experts who carried out the study, there is a higher incidence of children with genital malformations when parents are exposed to pesticides and polluting substances such as lead, hormones, plasticizers and drugs and these substances are also associated with the development of autism and intellectual disabilities. .

Andrey Rzhetsky, one of the researchers in charge and a member of the University of Chicago Medical Center, explains that autism seems to be strongly associated with the rate of male genital malformations in the United States, indicating that the problem stems from the environmental burden In other words, they are sure that the chemical substances mentioned have an effect on the development of microfalosomy.

Chapter 42. Cryptorchidism

Cryptorchidism is a genital problem that exclusively affects the male gender and is characterized by the incomplete descent of one or both testicles into the scrotum. Usually, the baby who presents it also suffers from an inguinal hernia.

The diagnosis of cryptorchidism is made by a physical examination by a pediatrician and sometimes a surgical intervention is necessary to remove the testicle that did not descend.

Normal development of the testicles in early stages

Normal testicular development in any male baby begins from the moment of conception and takes place in the retroperitoneal cavity of the fetus and then goes to the scrotal bag. The descent must occur between 28 and 40 weeks of gestation and is associated with hormonal and mechanical processes.

According to statistics, cryptorchidism affects about 3% of full-term newborns and up to 30% of newborns ahead of time. Two thirds of the undescended testicles before birth reach the scrotal bags spontaneously during the first 4 months of life. So 0.8% of babies require further treatment.

80% of cases of cryptorchidism are diagnosed clinically shortly after birth, the rest is done during childhood or early adolescence. The undescended testicle remains in the inguinal canal, along the path of descent, in the abdominal or retroperitoneal cavity near the kidneys, but this occurs less frequently.

Cryptorchidism can be unilateral when a single testicle does not descend or bilateral if both do not reach the scrotal pockets. Normally, only one of the testicles is affected but approximately 10% of cases affect both.

Why does cryptorchidism occur?

Testicular descent is conditioned by hormonal factors, for example, by androgens or Müllerian inhibition factor; physicists such as gubernulum regression and intra-abdominal pressure; and for maternal exposure to estrogenic or antiandrogenic substances.

Some conditions such as premature birth, restricted intrauterine growth, twin pregnancies and low birth weight can cause cryptorchidism in the baby, as well as gestational diabetes, some chromosomal abnormalities and the mother's advanced age.

Endocrine disruptors and cryptorchidism

To date, endocrine disruptors that are most associated with problems in the male reproductive system of the fetus are present in pesticides and to prove it a group of researchers from the nineties conducted an investigation.

The scientists started from the hypothesis that the substance with hormonal activity present in pesticides increases the risk of cryptorchidism, so they accounted for 270 cases of orchidopexy in children aged between 1 and 16 years.

Orchidopexy is the surgical intervention that requires cryptorchidism and the study was carried out at the Clinical Hospital of Granada. To make the study more specific, the researchers used the residence and health center as geographic units of reference for the analysis. With this data, a comparison was made.

In each region the rate of orchidopexy was estimated and this was compared with the use of pesticides, in this way they determined that the frequency of cryptorchidism increased in parallel with the use of pesticides in the different regions, with the exception of the capital of Granada.

At that time the researchers could not confirm a direct relationship between pesticides and the risk of cryptorchidism, but they did show a greater frequency of orchidopexy in children from municipalities near the Mediterranean coast, which is an area dedicated to intensive agriculture.

With early treatment in children you can experience normal growth of your genitals, be fertile when you reach reproductive age and reduce the risk of getting testicular cancer.

Chapter 43. Hypospadias

Hypospadias is an anomaly present only in men, when the penis manifests it does not develop in the usual way but the urinary meatus, which is the hole through which urine flows, is located in the lower part of the glans, in the trunk or at the junction of the scrotum and penis and not at the tip as it should.

This condition is anatomically due to incomplete closure of penile structures during embryogenesis, so the urethral opening moves along the ventral side of the limb and is not located towards the tip, so the child may experience difficulty urinating.

Abnormal urethra formation occurs between the 8th and 14th week of pregnancy and depending on its location the severity of the hypospadias varies, for example, 70% of cases the urethra is located below the glans or distally in the penis, these are considered mild, while only 30% of cases have a high severity.

How common is hypospadias?

In Europe approximately 18.6 births out of every 10,000 have this anomaly, while in North America the prevalence is higher and can be observed in 34.2 births out of every 10.0000.Asia is the continent with the lowest prevalence, since it barely reaches 0.69 of births by the mentioned figure.

Hypospadias is considered to be a mainly genetic anomaly because in 7% of cases there is at least one family member with the same problem, either first, second or third order and linked to his mother or father. The probability that the younger brother of a child with hypospadias is also affected is 17%.

What complications can it have?

When the urethra is near the glans it is a mild case, but as it approaches the scrotum it becomes more severe and both aesthetic and functional problems can occur. When hypospadias occurs with other malformations such as cryptorchidism, the fertility of the individual can be compromised.

In the most severe cases a twist of the trunk of the penis can be generated, which leads the head to a rotation and approach to the base, this generates that it is dysfunctional both for sexual intercourse and for urination.

In other patients the foreskin does not fully develop and forms a hood over the top of the glans, which is flat and tilted due to the narrow tissue that surrounds it. The result is a complete curvature of the male member.

Can it be generated by disruptors?

In various studies animals have been used and the effect of maternal exposure to synthetic estrogens has been evaluated to determine if it was an important factor in the appearance of hypospadias in the offspring, in most of these studies a positive result was obtained, however , thanks to the difference between those species and us, their effect on humans is still under discussion.

Another important hypothesis explains that some male reproductive disorders such as cryptorchidism, infertility and testicular cancer are interrelated with each other in a disorder called dysgenesis syndrome and also originates in the mother's exposure to estrogen during pregnancy.

For now, more evidence is needed to determine which chemicals can cause this condition in a fetus and to establish preventive guidelines. Given the relationship that exists among other diseases of the infantile male reproductive system, it is important to continue with the same forms of protection against the substance.

Chapter 44. Pubertal Gynecomastia

Pubertal gynecomastia, in simple terms, is the growth of the mammary glands in men during puberty. It is a transitory and benign situation that does not affect the health of the developing youth, only his appearance. In very few cases it represents a serious endocrine problem.

Gynecomastia can be unilateral, when a single breast grows or bilateral in case the development of breast tissue occurs in both and basically what the teenager experiences is the increase in the volume of tissue around the nipple, it can cause discomfort to the touch but does not exceed 4 cm.

Some men and boys suffering from obesity have fat in the chest area due to overweight, it is not breast development because it has a softer consistency and an irregular shape.

After three years the young man's body will return to normal. Usually no medications or surgery are prescribed, but attention should be paid to your endocrine health.

Because it happens?

As many men as women have breast tissue in the chest area, but only in females does it develop permanently during puberty and plays a role in reproduction.

In the male breast tissue there are estrogen and androgen receptors and the imbalance between these hormones is what generates gynecomastia. Estrogen stimulation and androgen inhibition induce breast growth. It is believed that the hormone leptin, present in fatty tissue, is involved in the development of breasts in men because it increases the activity of aromatase, an enzyme responsible for a fundamental step in the biosynthesis of estrogen.

Some non-obese men have high levels of leptin, which reinforces this theory. Approximately 50-60% of children develop transient gynecomastia at some stage of pubertal development, but it often occurs between ages 13 and 14. In 90% of cases, androgen levels reach adult levels and breast tissue undergoes an involution, this may merit from one to three years.

How do disruptors affect the appearance of breasts in young people?

A study by the National Institute of Environmental Health Sciences of North Carolina, United States, states that lavender and tree tea oil contain chemical agents that act as endocrine disruptors and that are largely responsible for breast tissue growth in teenagers

These two substances are present in bath soaps, body lotions, perfumes and laundry detergents and are normally used in oils to apply directly to the skin, because their influence on the endocrine system is little known.

The effect that lavender and tree tea have on the body is antiandrogenic, which means that it inhibits male hormones allowing the activity of female hormones, such as estrogen, for this reason a man could develop breasts, which is a female physical characteristic.

So far there is no evidence that other chemicals are responsible for gynecomastia and it is a temporary condition in men, just in case other abnormalities occur in their development becomes a real concern for the risk of your health.

Chapter 45. Male Infertility

A man is diagnosed as infertile when he has difficulty getting a woman pregnant after trying several times over a year.

This condition can revolve around low sperm production, abnormal functioning, or sperm transport ducts are blocked in some way. Certain injuries, diseases and lifestyle factors can decrease male fertility.

Most men do not perceive another symptom other than the difficulty of conceiving a child, but they may experience difficulty ejaculating, reduced sexual desire and erectile dysfunction.

Statistics indicate that in 40% of cases the infertility problem comes from the testicles and it is estimated that 1 in 20 men have a low number of sperm in the ejaculate and that 1 in 100 does not expel sperm in ejaculation. In 60% of patients there is no cause for their condition.

Male fertility

The fertility of the man and therefore his ability to get a woman pregnant is based on the quantity and quality of his sperm. If a man aspires to achieve a conception, he must:

- **Have healthy sperm:** At least one of your testicles must function properly and your body must produce adequate levels of testosterone.
- **Healthy seminal ducts:** Sperm is transported in semen and this mixture is conducted outside the penis in ejaculation. There should be no obstructions of any kind in these ducts.
- **The sperm must be functional:** A sperm must move (motility) quickly, if it does not reach the ovum or have the ability to penetrate it.
- **The amount of sperm should be adequate:** If the sperm count is low, the chances of conception are reduced. It must be above 39 million per ejaculation.

Male infertility and endocrine disruptors

Various substances are associated with male infertility, for example, polychlorinated biphenyls, pesticides, heavy metals and phthalates, which mainly affect androgens. Androgens are responsible for spermatogenesis and the development of male physical characteristics.

In rural areas, less sperm quality is observed compared to urban areas and many authors believe that this is due to the presence of endocrine disruptors in the pesticides used in the region. Other studies relate low testosterone levels to perfluorinated compounds.

On the other hand, PCBs can reduce semen quality by up to 50% and affect both the mobility and viability of sperm. The effect of this substance is one of the most worrisome, so much so that if 50 years were not prohibited, men could lose their ability to reproduce on their own.

Finally, there are heavy metals. In a study carried out in sterile couples that carried out their first IVF, sperm was analyzed in order to find biomarkers that could predict the outcome of this medical procedure but were not associated with sperm concentration, viability and mobility.

The researchers found that more than 40% of men were not exposed to lead for work reasons or smoked, however the concentration of this metal in the seminal and blood plasma exceeded the upper limit allowed and correlated inversely with the fertilization of the ovules .

In other words, when more lead was in the blood of the men in the lower experiment it was the ovulation rate, which triggered infertility.

In our society the rate of male infertility is alarming. For many specialists and health institutes, the fact that assisted motherhood is increasingly necessary is a cause for concern, is an indication that something is deeply affecting us and it is time to do something about it.

Chapter 46. Testicular Cancer

Testicular cancer is a type of abnormal cell growth that can develop in one or both testicles. It is a pathology that mainly affects young men, between the ages of 20 and 39.

Testicular cancer is common in men who had abnormal development during puberty, suffered cryptorchidism or have a family member who developed cancer. It is also usual in adults, only 6% of cases occur in children and adolescents and 8% in older adults.

World statistics indicate that in comparison with other cancer diseases, testicular cancer is rare, in fact, only 1 in 250 men will be affected at some point in their life.

For this year 2019, the American Cancer Society estimates that about 9,560 new cases will be diagnosed and that approximately 410 men will die from the disease.

In American men testicular cancer can appear from 15 years of age and more patients are reported below 35 years. Worldwide the average age of diagnosis is approximately 33 years.

Most of the time the disease is treated successfully, so the risk of a man dying of this cancer is 1 in 5,000, however the disease has doubled its incidence in recent decades.

What causes testicular cancer?

As with other similar pathologies, the exact causes of testicular cancer are not known, but scientists claim that it is closely related to other conditions such as cryptorchidism and that genes are also involved.

Most of the testicular cancer cells that have been observed have additional copies of a portion of chromosome 12, in other cases an abnormally high number of genetic material is observed and other tissues show modifications in chromosomes other than 12.

With this information, scientists cannot give definitive conclusions, but they got a common point to begin with.

Endocrine disruptors involved in the disease

Nor is there clear evidence that a specific group of endocrine disruptors promote the development of cancer in the testicles, but due to the increase in patients in recent years, scientists have little doubt that these are environmental factors.

At the University of Edinburgh, in Scotland, a group of scientists developed a model with which it is intended to demonstrate that embryonic exposure to phthalates exponentially increases the risk of developing testicular cancer between 20 and 40 years.

The team of researchers performed a tissue graft of aborted human fetuses under the skin of mice and in this model, the germ cells in the testicles are also in a critical state to know if there is any developmental failure that can make them pre - carcinogens.

Phthalate and other chemicals present around us considered harmless will be used and it will be observed if you predispose animals to develop cancer. For scientists this model has two limitations.

In the first place, it is a question whether the effect of phthalate on mice can be translated into humans and in the second, the life and development time of these animals is much shorter than ours, so the dynamics could be different.

This promising study aims to reach a conclusion that brings more knowledge about the disease and possible ways to avoid it.

Chapter 47. Prostate Cancer

Prostate cancer is a type of cancer that develops in the prostate. This gland is part of the male reproductive system, its shape is similar to that of a nut and is responsible for producing the seminal fluid that nourishes and transport sperm.

The prostate is just below the bladder, in front of the rectum and in its back coincides with the seminal vesicles, other glands that produce the most semen. The size of this gland changes over time, so in young people the prostate is smaller than in adult men and this modification is not due to any type of pathology.

The evolution of the patient diagnosed with prostate cancer does not follow a specific pattern. It usually grows slowly and is limited to the prostate gland, where it does not cause much damage, but in other patients the growth is accelerated and can spread rapidly. Early detection is more likely to be a successful treatment.

How common is it?

Prostate cancer is one of the most frequent among men, as is skin cancer. For this year it is estimated that the number of diagnoses will be 174,650 men in the United States, that 60% of the patients will be adults over 65 and that there will be 31,620 deaths due to this disease.

Globally, the average age of diagnosis is 66 years and the disease rarely occurs before age 40. In 90% of cases cancer is detected when it is limited to the prostate and adjacent organs, clinically this is called Local or regional stadium and is easier to deal with.

What causes prostate cancer?

The causes of this type of cancer are not clear, but the scientific information available to date relates it to genetics, ancestry, obesity and blood cholesterol levels.

For reasons not yet determined, men of African-American descent have a higher risk of suffering from the disease. Similarly, if there is a breast cancer survivor in the patient's family, the chances increase.

Obese men in general are at greater risk of prostate cancer due to high levels of cholesterol in their blood since this substance has an important role in the synthesis of androgens, estrogens and other active substances in the disease.

Cholesterol is the main element in the metabolism of lipids, the inflammatory response and other elements related to the formation and progression of cancer, therefore, when cholesterol is elevated, the risk increases.

Endocrine disruptors and prostate cancer

The action of endocrine disruptors is not fully defined despite the fact that various studies have been carried out. It is believed that fetal exposure to organochlorine pesticides such as chlorpyrifos and heavy metals such as arsenic plays an important role in the development of the disease in adulthood.

These two chemicals simulate the estrogen functions of the baby in formation and can profoundly alter it, so that it is more sensitive and prone to pathology a few decades later.

Both chlorpyrifos and arsenic are not currently banned and are supposedly used below legal and safe limits, but it is a questionable statement given the increase in the prevalence of the condition in recent years.

Chapter 48. Autism

"Autism" is the term that is generally used to refer to autism spectrum disorders. A person with autism is characterized by communication and social interaction problems, by presenting fixed interests, difficulty sharing and repetitive behaviors.

Autism spectrum disorders manifest in early childhood and persist throughout life, usually the diagnosis takes place before the first five years, because the child could also suffer from hyperactivity, attention deficit, epilepsy, anxiety and depression.

The intellectual level varies greatly among those affected, so a person with autism may have high cognitive skills and others instead of poor, but generally establish little eye contact, do not usually make social smiles and reject any type of physical contact.

Children and adults with autism spectrum disorders have tactile, olfactory, gustatory and auditory hypersensitivity, which helps maintain irritable behavior. They also have little pain sensitivity.

World statistics indicate that 1 out of every 160 children has an autism spectrum disorder and in Spain alone it is estimated that there are 450,000 people diagnosed. The prevalence of autism is higher in the male gender than in the female gender.

Indirect effect of endocrine disruptors

Direct exposure to a chemical does not cause autism spectrum disorder in the person, as it is a birth condition. The problem actually originates during pregnancy and is closely related to the mother's thyroid hormone levels.

Barbara Demeneix, author of the book "Toxic cocktail: how chemical pollution poisons our brains" and director of an important study that involved more than seven universities worldwide explains that exposure to various endocrine disruptors during pregnancy increases the risk of intellectual quotients low and neurological development disorders, such as autism.

The researchers who accompanied Demeneix shared with her the suspicion that the mixture of various substances in pregnancy had more weight than each one separately, so they used an epidemiological database composed of more than 2,300 pregnant women and created mixtures of chemicals similar to those that were exposed, in order to test them in laboratory animals.

Their findings were revealing, because they managed to achieve that concentrations similar to real life interfere with neural networks and in the expression of genes related to the autistic spectrum. They also found that the mixture of chemicals acts on the thyroid and on genes that regulate thyroid expression and this is essential for the development of fetuses.

In early embryonic stages the thyroid gland has not fully developed, so the fetus depends on the contribution of thyroid hormone from its mother. If she has a low level, there is no way to compensate for the lack and therefore the baby is at risk of autism and cognitive problems after birth.

This great contribution leaves a clue how harmful disruptors can be when they act together and how profound their impact is on our lives. Autism is a condition that is maintained from childhood to youth and is usually accompanied by other conditions that make the person's life more complex.

There is no cure for autism spectrum disorders, but the knowledge that the mother's hormones influence the development of the disorder gives us a clear route to prevent it.

Part IV Conclusions

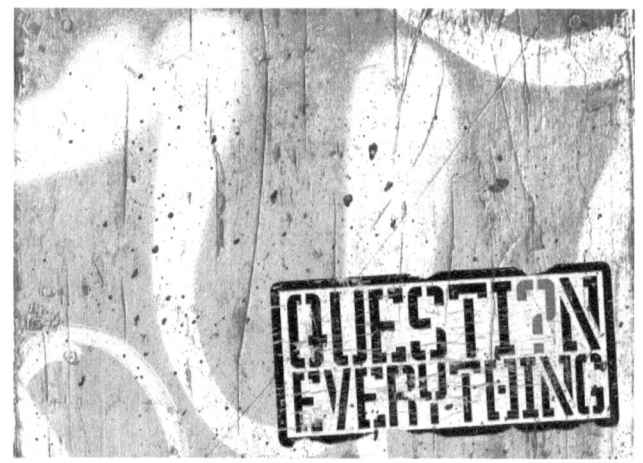

Chapter 49. My preventive recommendations to minimize pollution

As a specialist in Endocrinology and Family Medicine, my preventive recommendations to minimize contamination with endocrine disruptors are:

- Avoid old electrical equipment, remember that forty years ago PCBs were used in their manufacture.

- Prefer pesticide-free organic foods.

- Buy ecological cleaning utensils or companies that ensure user safety.

- Avoid dust, especially in children under three years of age.

- Wash new clothes before using them in order to remove chemical waste.

- Avoid dry and plasticized washings.

- Use mineral or vegetable based paints and always check that they are free of lead.

- Use digital thermometers instead of mercury thermometers.

- Take care of the consumption of fish and shellfish, always check their origin.
- Reduce the consumption of canned, plastic, hot food in plastic.

- Use microwave glass, not plastic.

- Do not expose plastic bottles to the sun.

- Avoid sun during harmful hours in order not to use sunscreens.

- Use nonylphenol-free gloves and detergents.

- Periodically replace toothbrushes, at least 3 times a year.

Epilogue

"SOS hormonal toxins" is a compilation of topics that address various aspects of chemical pollution of the environment and how these compounds have an impact on people's health status. The author, Dr. Mario Vega Carbó, clinical endocrinologist with more than 20 years of experience, organized in four sections and more than forty chapters, the main topics related to environmental chemical toxins that affect health, called endocrine disruptors.

The first part of the book presented in a chapter the basic concepts and generalities about endocrine disruptors. These are chemical substances, in general, that are products made by man and that stand out for presenting among their adverse effects direct alterations on the health of living beings, mainly affecting the function and regulation of the endocrine system, as well as they can cause embryonic development defects, genetic diseases and even neoplasms.

The second part of the book devoted each of its chapters to presenting the main toxic substances found in the environment, how is their elaboration process, how they get to have contact with people and what are the potential effects on health. In this section it was possible to recognize many compounds present in various objects that we use every day, for example, cleaning products, cosmetics, and even substances derived from insecticides and pesticides for the treatment of crops that arrive at our table in vegetables and fruits that we consume

In the third section he dealt with each of the diseases and clinical conditions that are related or that are influenced in their appearance, course and evolution by these toxins. The results of various studies and investigations that demonstrate the effects of endocrine disruptors on different organs and systems of the body were briefly discussed, leading to the development of pathological conditions.

The final section, by way of conclusion, presented a series of recommendations and guidelines aimed at offering resources to the reader to prevent such diseases and take care of their health.

We hope that the content of the text has served for your instruction; The purpose is always to educate the individual so that everyone can improve their health.

Thank you for purchasing and reading *SOS Hormonal Toxics!*

Bibliographic references

Bursian S., Newsted J., Zwiernik M. (2012). Polychlorinated biphenyls, polybrominated biphenyls, polychlorinated dibenzo-p-dioxins, and polychlorinated dibenzofurans. In: Ramesh C. Gupta (editor). Veterinary Toxicology Academic Press, Oxford, pp. 779-796.

Arlene Blum, Simona A. Balan, Martin Scheringer, Xenia Trier, Gretta Goldenman, Ian T. Cousins, Miriam Diamond, Tony Fletcher, Christopher Higgins, Avery E. Lindeman, Graham Peaslee, Pim de Voogt, Zhanyun Wang and Roland Weber (2015) The Madrid Statement on Poly- and Perfluoroalkyl Substances. Environmental Health Perspectives Vol. 123, No. 5

Ulla B. Mogensen, Philippe Grandjean, Flemming Nielsen, Pal Weihe and Esben Budtz-Jørgensen. "Breastfeeding as an Exposure Pathway for Perfluorinated Alkylates" Environmental Science & Technology August 20, 2015 doi: 10.1021 / acs.est.5b02237

Ecodes (2011) Perfluorinated compounds (PFCs) are in tap water and food, and affect health. ' Interview with Damià Barceló available at: https://ecodes.org/noticias/los-compuestos-perfluorados-pfcs-estan-en-el-agua-del-grifo-y-los-alimentos-y-afectan-la-salud # .Xa8DocfQjIU

Universidad de Las Palmas de Gran Canaria (2014) An expert in Toxicology at the ULPGC explains in El Mundo the effects of phthalates. Luis Domínguez interview available at: https://www.ulpgc.es/noticia/invesboada_20012014

AECOSAN (2013) Questions and answers about Bisphenol A. Original document available at: http://www.aecosan.msssi.gob.es/AECOSAN/docs/documento s/ food_security / risk_management / Questions_responses_bisphenol_A.pdf
Cosmetic Ingredient Review (2017) Safety Assessment of Parabens as Used in Cosmetics. Available at: https://www.cir-safety.org/sites/default/files/paraben _web.pdf

Guodong Zhang (2018) Triclosan, a Common Antimicrobial Ingredient in Toothpaste, Soaps, Linked to Colonic Inflammation, Altered Gut Microbiota. Available at: https://www.umass.edu/newsoffice/article/triclosan-common-antimicrobial-ingredient

P. D. Darbre, A. Aljarrah, W. R. Miller, N. G. Coldham, M. J. Sauer and G. S. Pope (2012) Concentrations of Parabens in Human Breast Tumors. KOURNAL OF APPLIED TOXICOLOGY J. Appl. Toxicol 24, 5–13 (2004) Published online in Wiley InterScience (www.interscience.wiley.com). DOI: 10.1002 / jat.958

Murali K. Matta, PhD1; Robbert Zusterzeel, MD, PhD, MPH1; Nageswara R. Pilli, PhD (2019) Effect of sunscreen application under maximal use conditions on plasma concentration of sunscreen active ingredients JAMA. 2019; 321 (21): 2082-2091. doi: 10.1001 / jama. 2019.5586

CA DownsEmail authorEsti Kramarsky-WinterRoee SegalJohn FauthSean KnutsonOmri BronsteinFrederic R. CinerRina JegerYona LichtenfeldCheryl M. WoodleyPaul PenningtonKelli Cadenas Contamination in Hawaii and the US Virgin Islands Archives of Environmental Contamination and Toxicology February 2016, Volume 70, Issue 2, pp 265–288

Cocca, Claudia; Ventura Clara; Nunez, Mariel; Randi, Andrea; Venturino, Andres (2015) Acta Toxicol. Argent. (2015) 23 (3): 142-152-142 -The organophosphorus chlorpyrifos as an estrogenic disruptor and risk factor for breast cancer. Toxicol Act. Argent. (2015) 23 (3): 142-152

De Waisbaum, R. G .; Rodriguez, Cristian RamonIcon; Sbarbati, Norma Ethel (2017) Determination of TBT in water and sediment samples along the Argentine Atlantic coast. Environmental Technology 0959-3330

David Santillo, Iryna Labunska, Maureen Fairley and Paul Johnston. Greenpeace (2003) Consuming chemistry. An electronic version of this report is available on the website: www.greenpeace.org/espana_es/

Catherine E Rice, Kim Van Naarden Braun, Michael D Kogan, Camille Smith (2007) Screening for Developmental Delays Among Young Children --- National Survey of Children's Health, United States. Available at: https://www.researchgate.net/publication/265516534_Screeni ng_for_Developmental_Delays_Among_Young_Children_---_National_Survey_of_Children's_Health_United_States_2007

Soler-Blasco R, Murcia M, Lozano M, Aguinagalde X, Iriarte G, Lopez-Espinosa MJ, Vioque J, Iñiguez C, Ballester F, Llop S. Exposure to mercury among 9-year-old Spanish children: Associated factors and trend throughout childhood. Environ Int. 2019 Jun 18; 130: 104835. doi: 10.1016 / j.envint. 2019.05.029. [Epub ahead of print]. PMID: 31226565

European Association for the Study of Diabetes (2015) Pesticide exposure is related to the risk of diabetes. European

Association for the Study of Diabetes, news release, Sept. 15, 2015

Department of Analytical Chemistry The Connecticut Agricultural Experiment Station (2012) Removal of Trace Pesticide Residues from Produce. Available at: https://portal.ct.gov/CAES/Fact-Sheets/Analytical-Chemistry/Removal-of-Trace-Pesticide-Residues-from-Produce

Tianxi Yang, Orcid Jeffrey Doherty, Bin Zhao, Amanda J. Kinchla, John M. Clark, Lili He Effectiveness of Commercial and Homemade Washing Agents in Removing Pesticide Residues on and in Apples. J. Agric. Food Chem. 201765449744-9752
Ángel Nadal (2012) Endocrine disruptors. Available at: http://dspace.umh.es/bitstream/11000/4649/1/Ángel%20Nadal.pdf

Ángela L. Londoño, Beatriz Restrepo, Juan F. Sánchez, Alejandro García-Ríos, Adolfo Bayona and Patricia Landázuri Pesticides and hypothyroidism in farmers in banana and coffee growing areas, in Quindío, Colombia. Rev. Public Health. 20 (2): 215-220, 2018

Rzhetsky A, Bagley SC, Wang K, Lyttle CS, Cook EH Jr, et al. (2014) Environmental and State-Level Regulatory Factors Affect the Incidence of Autism and Intellectual Disability. PLoS Comput Biol 10 (3): e1003518. doi: 10.1371 / journal.pcbi.1003518

Barbara A Cohn, Piera M Cirillo, Mary Beth Terry (2019) DDT and Breast Cancer: Prospective Study of Induction Time and Susceptibility Windows. Journal of the National Cancer

Institute, Volume 111, Issue 8, August 2019, Pages 803–810, https://doi.org/10.1093/jnci/djy198

Leonardo Trasande (2016) Women's chemical exposure may cost Europe more than $ 1 billion. Journal of Clinical Endocrinology and Metabolism, online March 22, 2016.

Laura Birks, Maribel Casas, Ana M. Garcia, Jan Alexander, Henrique Barros, Anna Bergström, Jens Peter Bonde, Alex Burdorf, Nathalie Costet, Asta Danileviciute, Merete Eggesbø, Mariana F. Fernández, M. Carmen González-Galarzo, Regina Gražulevičienė , Wojciech Hanke, Vincent Jaddoe, Manolis Kogevinas, Inger Kull, Aitana Lertxundi, Vasiliki Melaki (2016) Occupational Exposure to Endocrine-Disrupting Chemicals and Birth Weight and Length of Gestation: A European Meta-Analysis. Environmental Health Perspectives Vol. 124, No. 11

John Meeker (2018) Phthalate exposure linked to preterm birth. Available at: https://news.umich.edu/phthalate-exposure-linked-to-preterm-birth/
Andrey Rzhetsky, Steven C. Bagley, Kanix Wang, Christopher S. Lyttle, Edwin H. Cook Jr, Russ B. Altman, Robert D. Gibbons (2014) Environmental and State-Level Regulatory Factors Affect the Incidence of Autism and Intellectual Disability. Available at: https://journals.plos.org/ploscompbiol/article?id=10.1371/jour na l.pcbi.1003518

Mariana F. Fernández, Begoña Olmos, Nicolás Olea (2012) Exposure to endocrine disruptors and alterations of the male urogenital tract (cryptorchidism and hypospadias) Available at: https://www.scielosp.org/article/gs/2007.v21n6/500 -514 /

Ramsey J, Li Y, Arao Y, Naidu A, Coons LA, Diaz A, Korach KS (2019) Lavender Products Associated With Premature Thelarche and Prepubertal Gynecomastia: Case Reports and Endocrine-Disrupting Chemical Activities J Clin Endocrinol Metab. 2019 Nov 1; 104 (11): 5393-5405.

European Society of Human Reproduction and Embryology (2010) Scientists develop the first model for investigating the origins of testicular cancer in humans. Available at: https://www.sciencedaily.com/releases/2010/08/10080320044 3.htm
Jaime Mendiola a, Jorge Ten a, Fernando Araico b, Carmen Martín Ondarza b, Alberto M Torres-Cantero c, José M Moreno-Grau d, Stella Moreno-Grau d, Rafael Bernabeu (2007) Rev Int Androl. 2007; 5: 173-80

About the author:

Dr. Mario Vega Carbó

- The Cuban doctor graduated in 1994.
- Specialist in endocrinology and family medicine.
- Master in longevity and ultrasound.
- Professor of Medical Pathophysiology.
- Lovers of good, family and nature.

Other books

1. An approach to natural endocrinology
2. Endocrine alarms: save lives
3. ABC of the endocrinologist for the layperson
4. Recipes for your hormone
5. Where Queen of Hormones ... short stories
6. Food myths, vision of the endocrinologist
7. S.O. Hormone toxins, naked truths
8. Vitamin D: an omnipresent hormone?
9. Hormones, exercises and fitness bodies
10. Obesity, diabetes, thyroid and S.O.P.

Available in 10 languages!

Social media

 drvegaendocrino.com Dr. Mario Vega - Tu Endocrino Online

 @drvegaendocrino @drmariovegaendocrinologo

Synopsis

We live with them daily, they are present in the air, on the ground, in the water, in food, in cleaning and personal hygiene products. We are talking about endocrine disruptors, chemical substances produced by man, that alter the function of the endocrine system and consequently, the processes of our body regulated by hormones.

SOS Hormonal toxics, is another of the works of Dr. Mario Vega Carbó, a specialist in endocrinology, who brings this opportunity a text oriented to educate about the risks derived from chemical pollution of the environment, with a simple and clear language for all audiences.

The text is divided into four main sections that explain the generalities and basic information of neuroendocrine disruptors, their classification and composition, where these toxic substances are found, how they interact with the environment, and their impact on people's health.

The book details the main diseases and pathological conditions that are related to endocrine disruptors, supporting this information in the results of scientific studies carried out in prestigious universities.

We invite you to enjoy this reading and learn more about the chemicals around us, their toxicity, consequences and prevention.

Dedication

To the health of my wife Ethel Delfa Vado Osuna
To the health of my children, grandchildren and their
descendants:
Liuba Lucia Vega Vado
Fidel Ernesto Vega Carbó
Mario Enrique Vega Carbó
Rocio Vega Suarez
For the current and future health of the human race